THAI TABLE MASSAGE

BY ELEFTERIA MANTZOROU

Copyright © 2018 by Eleftheria Mantzorou.

Elefteria Mantzorou
Flow.heavenly@gmail.com
Jointheflow.weebly.com

Although the author and publisher have made every effort to ensure that the information in this book was correct at press time, the author and publisher do not assume and hereby disclaim any liability to any party for any loss, damage, or disruption caused by errors or omissions, whether such errors or omissions result from negligence, accident, or any other cause.

This book is not intended as a substitute for the medical advice of physicians. The reader should regularly consult a physician in matters relating to his/her health and particularly with respect to any symptoms that may require diagnosis or medical attention.

Contents

Introduction

In this book we will see how we can apply the techniques of traditional Thai Massage, which is performed on the floor, on the massage table. I have focused on techniques that do not require the therapist to ascend fully on the table, as this has little difference from applying the techniques on the floor. The experienced Thai Massage therapists will see that I have omitted some typical techniques, as their application is difficult or ineffective on the table.

On the other hand, I present some other techniques, which have a similar effect on the body, with those that are performed on the floor.

The receiver is dressed, as in traditional Thai Massage.

I demonstrate the techniques according to the protocol of traditional Thai Massage. That is, I will start in supine position, then I will proceed to the side position, then to prone position, and finally to the face. I start from the feet, and proceed towards the head, in all positions. At some points, you will hear me saying that I am working on the sen lines. This is a process called "Jap Sen" in Thai.

What is Thai Table Massage?

Thai Table Massage is not a traditional modality, as there were no massage tables in Thailand until the recent decades. Thai Massage, an ancient form of bodywork, is traditionally practiced on the floor. And as we will see, most of its techniques can be applied successfully on the table, sometimes with some modifications.

Thus, Thai Table Massage is Thai Massage work performed on the table. You can combine it with any modality, or perform it by itself.

One consideration, which is often overlooked in traditional Thai Massage, is the range of motion during the application of the techniques. You should not overdo it, as this may cause harm. Less is more, in most of cases.

Work on the table vs. work on the floor

When we work on the floor, we have the advantage of being on the same level with our client. This allows us to use more efficiently our bodyweight. A small sized person will be able to apply the Thai Massage leverages and locks more easily on the floor. The disadvantage is that work on the floor usually takes its toll on the therapist's lower back and knees.

On the other hand, work on the table is much more comfortable for the therapist's back and knees. However, on the table we access the client in considerably different angles, and that can have an impact on the efficiency of some techniques - especially of those that require strength, in addition to skill.

Ultimately, the choice to work on the table or on the floor, is up to the therapist. The core traditional Thai Massage work, that includes Jap Sen (work on the Thai meridians), Tok Sen (tapping with wooden tools), and Luk Pra Kob (herbal compress) can definitely be performed on the table. Moreover, since the client is placed on the table, it is possible to combine Thai Massage techniques with work from other modalities, like Swedish massage, manual therapy, osteopathy, structural integration, etc.

Combining Thai Table Massage and Swedish massage

One of the most important features of Thai Massage, is that it is a dry form of bodywork. The client always wears light clothes during a Thai Massage session, so that the therapist can maintain a stable hold of the extremities, the torso and the joints during manipulation.

On the other hand, Swedish massage is performed with oil, and directly on the skin. How do you combine these two modalities?

First of all, determine the client's goals and needs, since many people who come for a Swedish massage are looking for relaxation and do not wish to respond to verbal instructions like "hold my hand", "lift your leg", or instructions about breathing. Many people who come for a massage, just want to let go. Thus, many of the Thai Table techniques will not be suitable for these people. You can still apply some Thai Table techniques however, that do not involve instructions or lifting extremities.

Obviously, in such a combination, the client should be undressed, but of course covered with towels and / or sheets. You will definitely need a very large towel or sheet in order to apply the Thai Table manipulations.

This is how I do it: Start with Swedish massage, in order to warm the tissues, and then cover the client properly. This is necessary in order to maintain the client's dignity, to keep the body warm, and to meet possible legal requirements (each country or state may have its own regulations - be sure to know them well). Apply the manipulations that are desirable, and then continue with Swedish massage techniques.

Sip Sen – The Ten Lines

In the Thai language, sen means "line". The Thai meridians are called Sen, and in massage therapy, ten basic "lines" are used (sip means "ten").

The sen have more similarities with the Ayurvedic nadi, than with the Chinese meridians. The sen do not correspond to specific organs, like the Chinese meridians, and are indicated for problems that may occur across their course. Each sen has some acupressure points.

Sen work is called jap sen, and it is done in 5 steps:

- Stretching (opening the line)
- Walking with palms (warming the line)
- Walking with thumbs (working on specific lines and points)
- Walking with palms (warming the line)
- Stretch (opening the line).

According to the traditional protocol, the therapist should start working upwards all sen lines – that is, from the feet towards the head, and from the hands towards the heart. Then, he should return to the starting point. Bear in mind that there may be some differences to this protocol, depending on the school.

It is not necessary to work all the lines in one session, and it is not necessary to work on the whole course of a line.

Jap sen should be applied after training with a qualified teacher.

There are many sen lines crossing the legs. There are three lines on the outer surface of the leg, and 3 in the interior.

These are the lines that run on the outer leg:

1st line: Itha or Pingkala
2nd line: Sahatsarangsi or Tawaree
3rd line: Itha or Pingkala

These are the lines that run on the inner leg:

1st line: Sahatsarangsi or Tawaree
2nd line: Kalatharee
3rd line: Itha or Pingkala

My instructors in Thailand used to say that a Sen line can have one of three colors: white (corresponds to nerves), red (corresponds to arteries), or black (corresponds to veins).

Work on the Sen lines can be used to "open" deeper levels of the body. According to Thai medicine, the human body has five levels:

1. Epidermis (the top layer of the skin).
2. Subcutaneous tissue (also known as the hypodermis or superficial fascia).
3. Sen lines
4. Bones
5. Organs

Now, let's have a look at the Sen lines – the Thai meridians.

1, 2. Itha & Pingkala sen

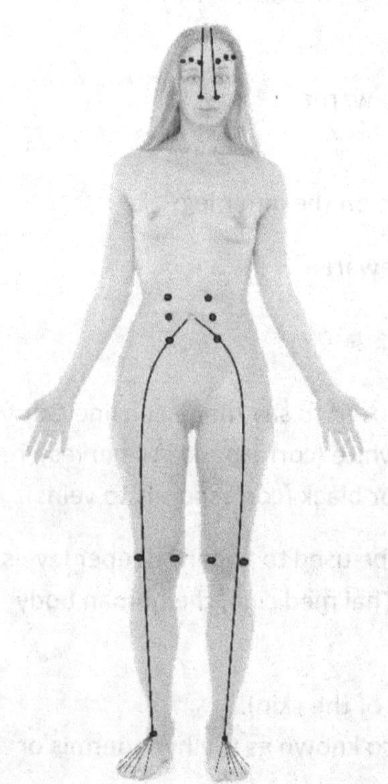

Itha originates from the navel and descends the anterior part of the left thigh, forming the first external line. Then it turns outwards on the left knee, and then follows an upward course between the heads of the posterior thigh muscles, forming the third inner line. It continues its course next to the spine, passes from the scalp and the forehead, and finally ends on the left nostril.

Pingkala follows the same path, but on the right part of the body.

These meridians also have sub-branches.

There is a sub-branch that continues until the toes of the dorsal aspect of the foot, and another that run between the heads of the gastrocnemius muscle (starts below the knee joint).

Also, in the upper part of the thoracic spine, there is another sub-branch, which passes next to the scapula, crosses the anterior surface of the arm and the dorsal surface of the hand, and ends on the fingertips.

Finally, there is a sub-branch above each eyebrow.

Another sub-branch starts from the hip bone and runs down to the ankle, forming the third outer energy line of the leg.

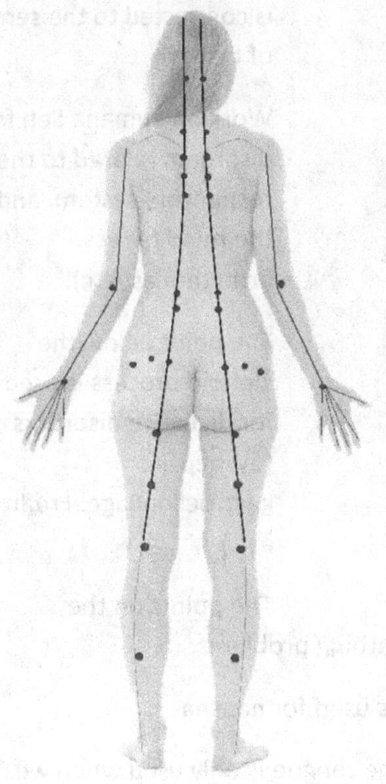

Work on the Itha and Pingkala for these problems:

- Muscle aches (back pain, sciatica, neck pain).
- Pain in the knee joint.
- Carpal tunnel syndrome (work on the arm points shown on the photo).
- Sinusitis (work the points on the face).
- The six points on the belly are used for digestive problems (refer to the section of abdominal techniques for the procedure), and for lower back pain.

These sen are connected to the sense of smell.

3. Sumana Sen

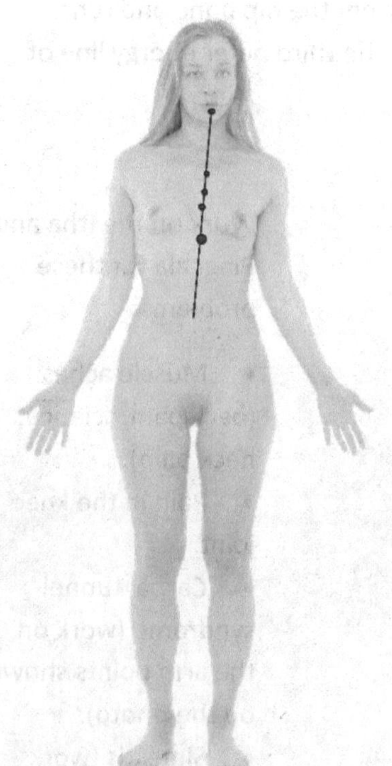

Sumana Sen originates from the navel, crosses the trunk, and ends at the root of the tongue. It is connected to the sense of taste.

Work on Sumana Sen for disorders related to the respiratory system, and the mind (stress, arrhythmias, etc).

The point below the xiphoid process is used for digestive disorders (dyspepsia, gastroesophageal reflux, etc.)

The points on the sternum are used for breathing problems.

The point below the lips is used for nausea.

The point at the root of the tongue is only used when we want to eliminate some toxic substance from the body via emesis. In order to activate it, the finger is inserted into the oral cavity (needless to say, never do this at a client!).

4. Kalatharee Sen

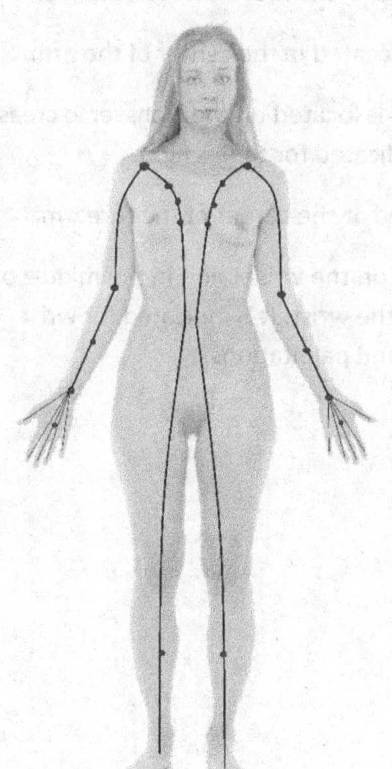

Kalatharee Sen originates from the navel and is divided into four major branches: two branches descend on the trunk, run on the legs (forming the second inner line) and end at the toes, on the plantar surface.

The other two branches run upwards on the trunk, cross the arm (between the ulna and radius) and end on the fingertips, on the palmar surface.

Kalatharee Sen is used for problems in the arms and legs (pain, weakness, numbness, muscle aches, etc.). However, it is also the main sen indicated for arrhythmias and disorders of the nervous system.

Kalatharee Sen is connected to the sense of touch.

The points of the legs are shown in the illustration.

One is located three fingers below the knee, while the other is next to the ankle.

Points on the arms and hands:

The first point of the arm is lateral and superior to the sternum at the lateral side of the first intercostal space.

There is a second point, located in the center of the arm.

The third point is located is located on the transverse crease of the elbow, and it is indicated for tennis elbow.

The fourth point is located at the center of the forearm.

There is also a fifth point on the wrist joint, in the middle of the transverse crease of the wrist. It is indicated for wrist pain, and also for stress and palpitations.

5, 6. Sahatsarangsi & Tawaree Sen

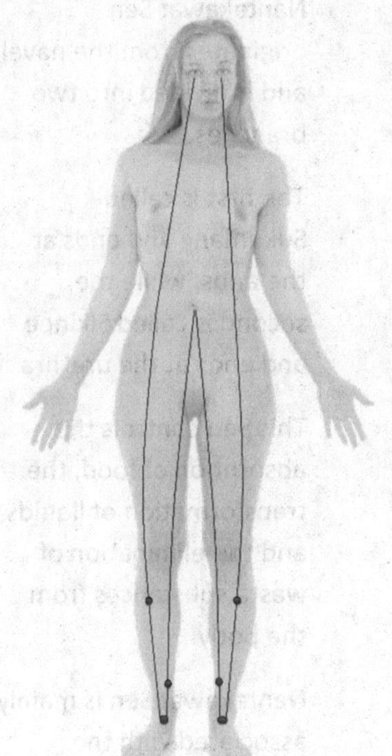

Sahatsarangsi Sen originates from the navel, descends at the inner surface of the left leg, forming the first inner line. Then it turns on the left ankle, forming the second outer line, and runs upwards to the neck. It ends below the left eye.

Tawaree Sen follows the same path, but on the right part of the body.

Both Sen are connected to the sense of sight.

These two sen are used for leg and eye problems. If there is an eye problem, work on the sen that runs on the opposite leg (e.g. if there is a problem on the left eye, work on Tawaree sen).

The first point is located is located four finger widths down from the bottom of the patella, along the outer boundary of the shin bone. Use it for pain on the legs.

The second point is on the dorsum of the foot, at the midpoint of the transverse crease of the ankle joint. It is indicated for ankle pain.

7. Nantakawat Sen

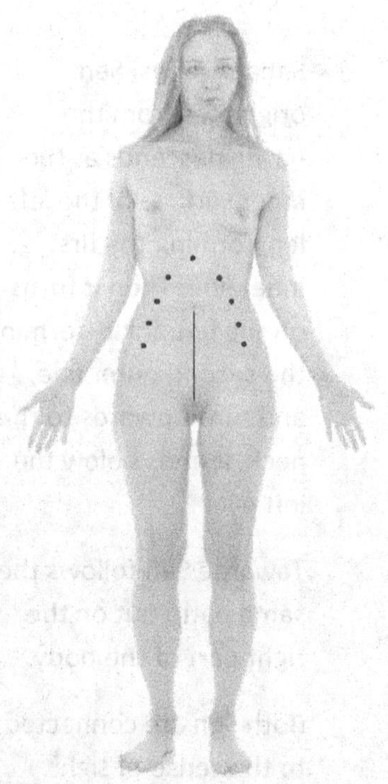

Nantakawat Sen originates from the navel and is divided into two branches.

The first is called Sukumang and ends at the anus, while the second is called Sikinee and ends at the urethra.

This Sen controls the absorption of food, the transformation of liquids and the elimination of waste substances from the body.

Nantakawat Sen is mainly associated with the processes of urination and defacation.

Generally, it is used for digestive problems (constipation, irritable bowel syndrome, etc.).

In cases of constipation work in a clockwise direction, while in cases of diarrhea work anticlockwise, on the 9 points shown on the illustration.

8, 9. Lawusang & Ulanga Sen

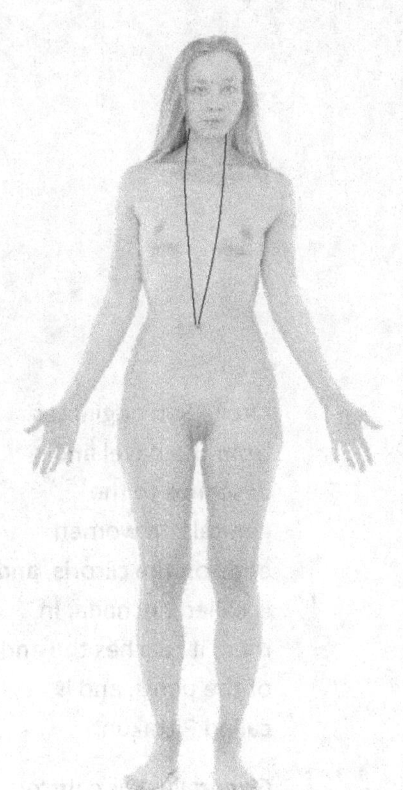

These two Sen have two alternative names in the Thai language. Lawusang is also called Chantapusang, while the Ulanga sen is also called Luchang.

Lawusang Sen originates from the navel, runs upwards on the trunk, passes next to the left ear, and ends on the temples.

Ulanga Sen follows the same path, but on the right side of the body. These two Sen control the sense of hearing.

Generally, they are used for pain on the face. They can be used for:

- earache and tinnitus (due to stress).
- any pain not due to acute inflammation (e.g. headaches).
- motion sickness.

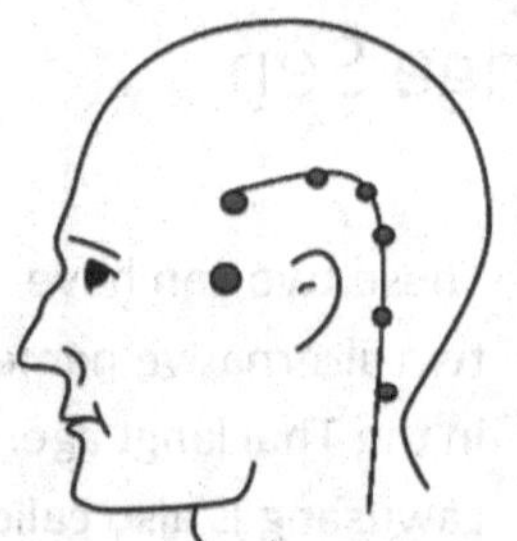

The course of Lawusang and Ulanga Sen around the ear.

10. Kitcha Sen

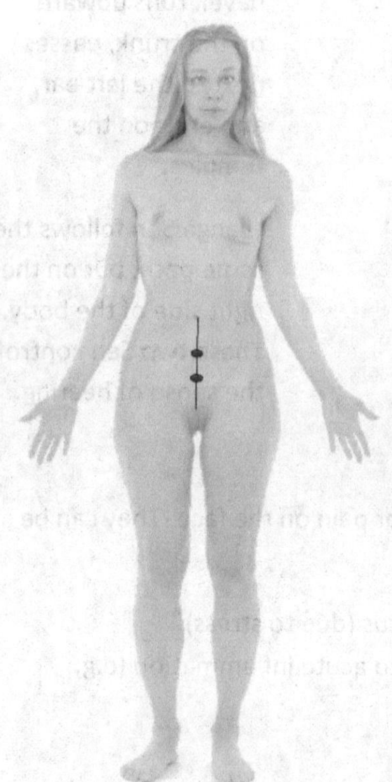

Kitcha Sen originates from the navel and descends to the genitals. In women ends on the clitoris, and is called Kitchana. In men, it reaches the end of the penis, and is called Pittakun.

Generally, it is controls sexual arousal, and reproductive capacity and function. Kitcha Sen is used mainly in cases of sexual frigidity, erectile dysfunction, and also for disorders of the female reproductive system.

Method of working

Thai Table Massage (like Thai Massage) is best done slowly and deeply. If you work quickly, the parasympathetic nervous system will not relax, and the receiver's body will not "assimilate" properly your work. Speed definitely plays an important role.

Palm and thumb walking

Thus, palm walking, presses and thumb walking should be applied for 3-5 seconds EACH time. Moreover, you should press gradually, and simultaneously inspect and "listen" to the tissues. Never go beyond the limit that is naturally set from the receiver's body.

Palm and / or thumb walking and pressing can be used interchangeably in this book, and they are synonyms.

Stretching

Hold all stretches for 5-10 seconds, and repeat 2-3 times. The first time you apply a stretch, inspect the range of motion. Then, the second time, you can go a little further. In any case, respect the body's boundaries. Whenever you apply intense stretches - especially those that involve lifting the extremities - be sure to warm the muscles and the tissues before that, otherwise injuries may occur.

I have found out that professional dancers, yoga and Pilates teachers and dedicated practitioners do not need a lot of stretching in a Thai Massage (or Table) session, because they are anyway doing a lot of stretching themselves. These people need more thumb and palm walking, and focused work on the muscles.

Joint rotation

I am very well aware of the fact that modern conventional physiotherapy forbids joint rotation. I was taught to apply joint rotations in my Thai Massage training, and I still apply it, although gently. Whenever you rotate a joint, be attentive for any "sounds" within the joint - these may mean that the ligaments that support this joint, are now loose. Thus, in that case, you should not pull forcibly that joint.

Joint rotation can be used to increase the range of motion. Please be aware of this: all mobilizations are at the same time diagnostic tools.

Acupressure

All points should be pressed or rubbed for 10 seconds, 3 times. It is better to do acupressure when working upwards on a sen line.

Breathing

When performing mobilizations, it is a good idea to synchronize your breathing with the client's breathing. It is recommended to perform the stretching or the manipulation upon exhalation (this is very important in abdominal work, where pressing should be done only upon exhalation). However, if a client is too stressed and his/her breathing is shallow and quick, the therapist should not follow this pattern!

If you do practice synchronized breathing, listen to the client's breath, and keep verbal instructions to a minimum.

Choosing a massage table

Thai Table massage can be performed on a usual massage table. You do not need a hydraulic table, although it is always an advantage to have one when performing manipulations and mobilizations that call for height adjustments.

As for its height, I personally keep it to the height I use for Swedish massage. In order to find the ideal height of the massage table for you, stand next to the table. The table should reach the first knuckle of your index finger. You should lower your table if you are working on a larger client.

The width of the table should be large enough, so that the client feels comfortable, but not too large, because then the therapist will have to bend forwards in order to reach and mobilize the client's body.

Contraindications & precautions

Although beneficial for many problems, Thai Table Massage has the following contraindications.

• Thai Table Massage is contraindicated if the receiver has fever or any infectious disease.

• Do not exert pressure on inflammatory areas (e.g. with dermatitis or eczema).

• Thai Table Massage is contraindicated if there aneurysm, thrombophlebitis or any other serious cardiovascular disease.

• If the patient is suffering from cancer, we can work very mildly. Sen work is usually safe. Applying more dynamic techniques is possible only after at least 3 months after chemotherapy or radiotherapy. In any case, the consent of the oncologist is necessary.

• Thai Table Massage is contraindicated to clients with osteoporotic fractures (and any fracture that has not healed properly). This applies topically.

• Thai Table Massage is not recommended during pregnancy, at least during the first trimester. After that, it is possible to apply some techniques, especially those of the side position. Avoid any deep work and pressure on the legs.

• Thai Table Massage is contraindicated in people who have undergone organ transplantation. Thai Table Massage (in fact, any form of bodywork) may boost the immune system, and can therefore be harmful in this case.

• If the receiver has any health problem that raises doubts as to whether Thai Table Massage is suitable for that person, a doctor should be consulted.

• Always respect the receiver's physical limitations. Avoid strong back bends in all people.

Massage space & hygiene

Here are some rules for the area where the Thai Table massage is performed:

• Thai Table Massage requires more space than classic Swedish massage, because of its stretches.

• Have at least 3-4 pillows to support the body of the receiver correctly.

• The therapist and the receiver should wear comfortable, loose clothes.

• The room must be very clean.

• I recommend dim lighting and soothing music.

• The receiver should not have eaten a heavy meal at least two hours before a Thai Table Massage session. After the session, I tell my clients to avoid food for the next hour, to drink lots of water, and to bathe after 2-3 hours.

• The therapist should wash his hands before the massage.

• The massage table should be cleaned with antiseptic soap, spray or steam after each session. Sheets should be washed with hot water and soap.

Now let' see some techniques of Thai Table Massage.

Supine position

The supine position is good for leg pain, as well as for lower back pain, as it contains stretches for the muscles that support the pelvis. From this position, you can also work on the belly, the chest and the arms.

Props are recommended. That is, it is recommended to place a pillow under the knees and under the head, when we are working on the torso, the arms and the face. However, the feet and leg techniques include many mobilizations and thus a pillow under the knees is useless. You can, of course, place a pillow under the knees when you complete all the techniques for the legs, and proceed to the torso.

Now, let's see how you can apply the traditional Thai Massage techniques on the table. We will start from the feet, as in traditional Thai Massage.

These techniques warm the feet and the legs, and prepare the body for the more dynamic work that comes after that. They are also considered suitable for the treatment of plantar fasciitis (during the chronic phase). Other traditional indications include painful, tired feet, headaches and stress.

The feet

Techniques for the feet

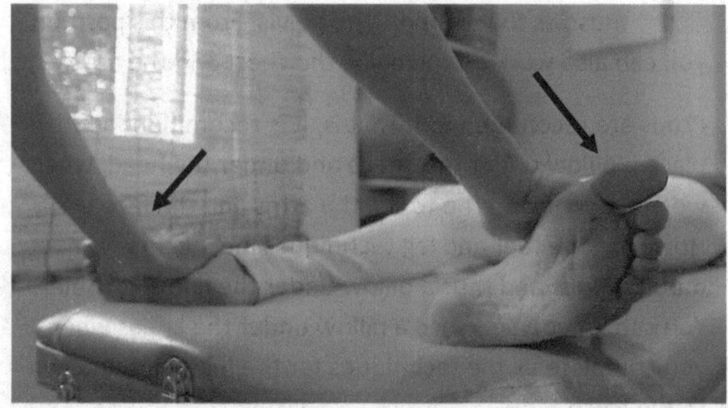

1. Press alternatively on the inner arch of the foot. Press on 2-3 spots, depending on the length of the arch. Avoid pressing on the ball of the foot. The angle of pressure should be about 45 degrees. Repeat 10 times on each foot.

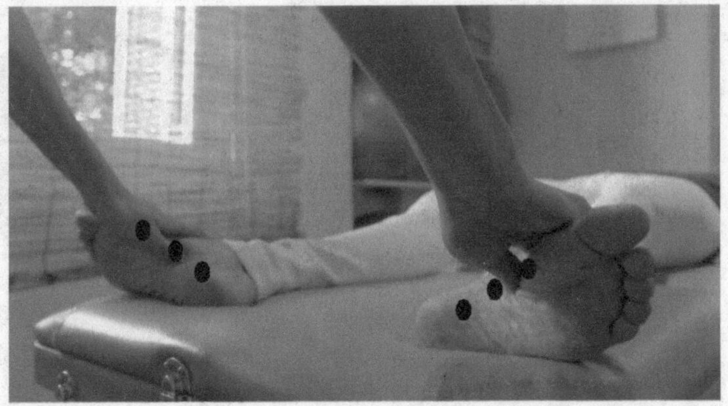

2. Press 3-4 spots on the inner arch of the foot. Rub the spot, and then press for 3 seconds, on each spot. Learn to "listen" to the receiver's body, and do not press more than the extent that the body allows.

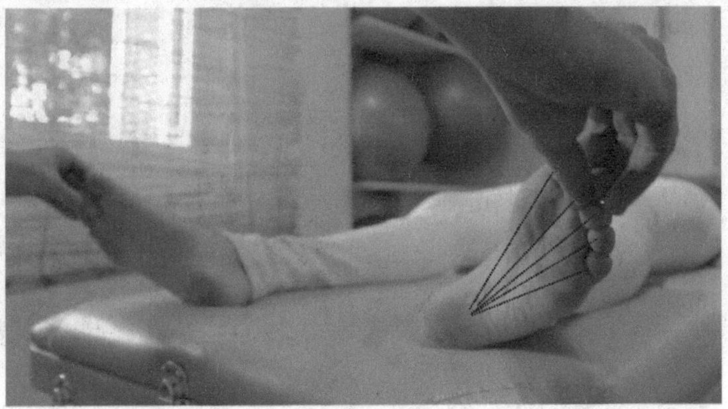

3. Work on the Kalatharee Sen branch of the foot. This consists of five lines, each ending on a toe.

Work simultaneously, on both feet. At the end of each "line", pull gently the toe.

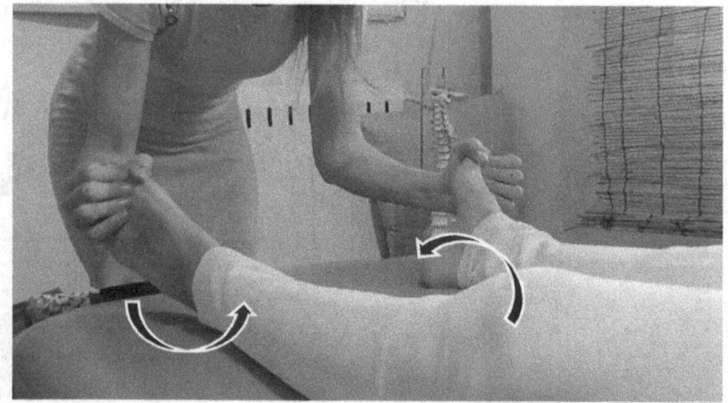

4. Grasp the feet, and rotate them. Your grip should not be too tight, but it should be firm. The feet should be open, at the width of the shoulders.

Do five rotations at both directions. Work slowly, and listen for possible "sounds" in the joint, that may point to loose ligaments.

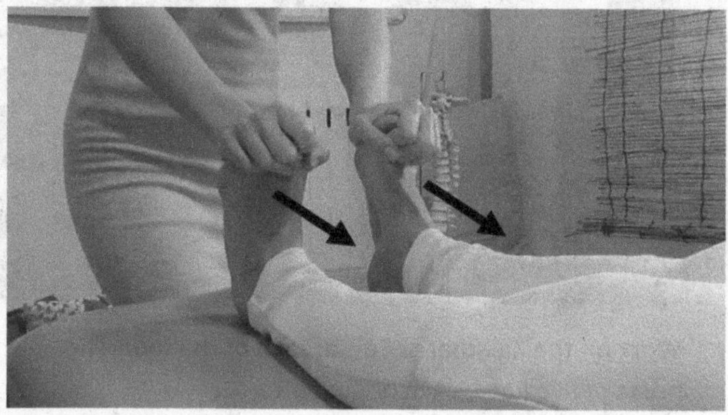

5. Maintaining the previous grip, bring the feet close to each other, in order to align them with the sagittal plane of the body. Push the feet upwards, and hold the stretch for 5-10 seconds. Repeat 3 times. The stretch should be felt on the Achilles tendon.

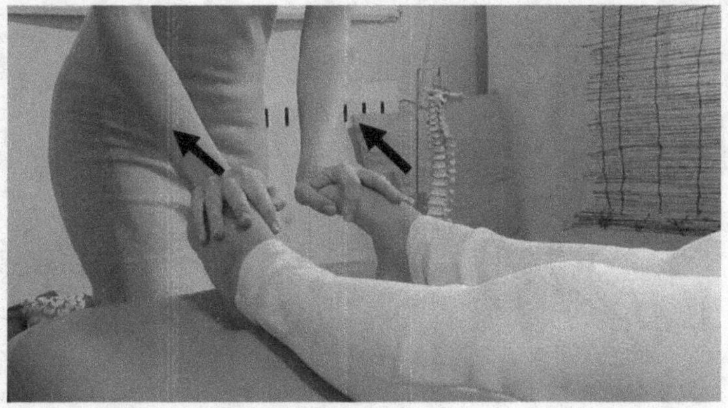

6. Maintaining the previous grip, and with the feet still close to each other, and aligned with the sagittal plane of the body, pull the feet downwards. Hold the stretch for 5-10 seconds. Repeat 3 times. The stretch should be felt on the muscles in the anterior compartment of the lower leg.

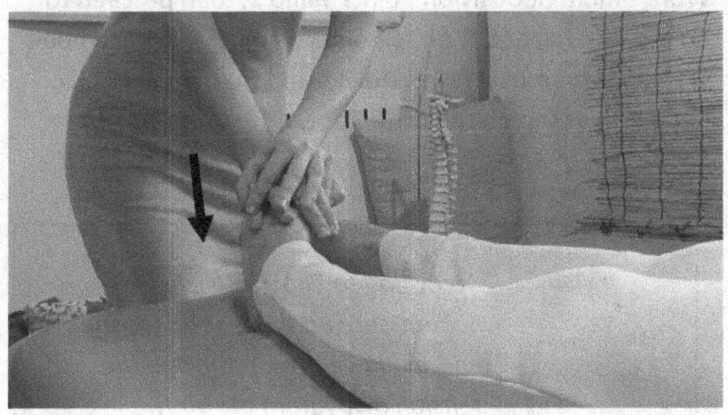

7. Cross the feet and press them. Hold the stretch for 5-10 seconds. Repeat 3 times. Omit this in osteoporotic women, and in people who are not flexible enough for this technique.

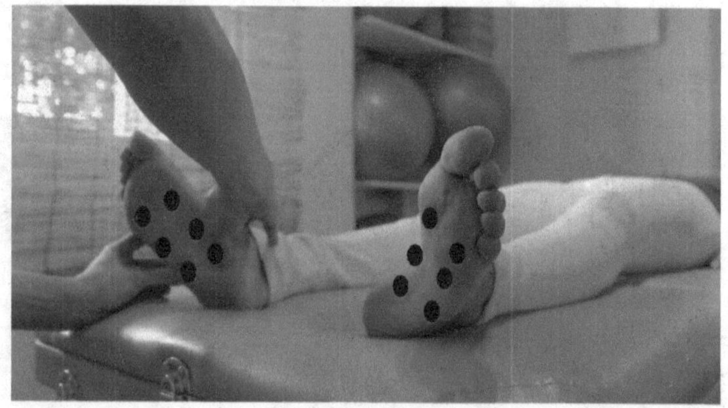

8. Work on six points on the plantar aspect of each foot. Work on each foot separately.

Points 1 and 2 are below the level of the ball of the foot, points 3 and 4 are at the level of the transverse arch, and points 5 and 6 are just above the level of the heel.

Work simultaneously on points 1 and 2, then proceed to points 3 and 4, and then to points 5 and 6. Rub each point with your thumbs 3 times slowly, and then press gently. Repeat this step on the other foot.

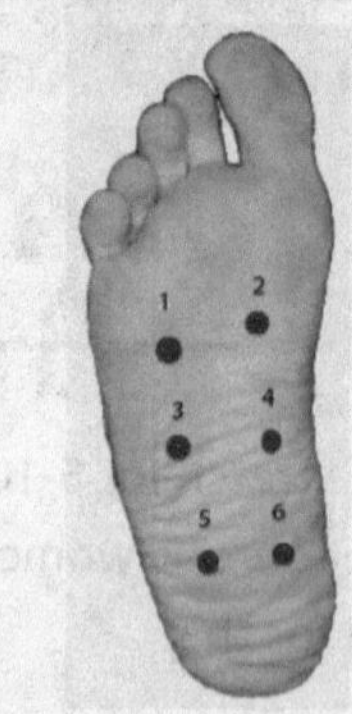

According to Thai medicine, acupressure on the feet brings the energy down, thus removing the tension away from the body.

For this reason, this technique is especially indicated for headaches.

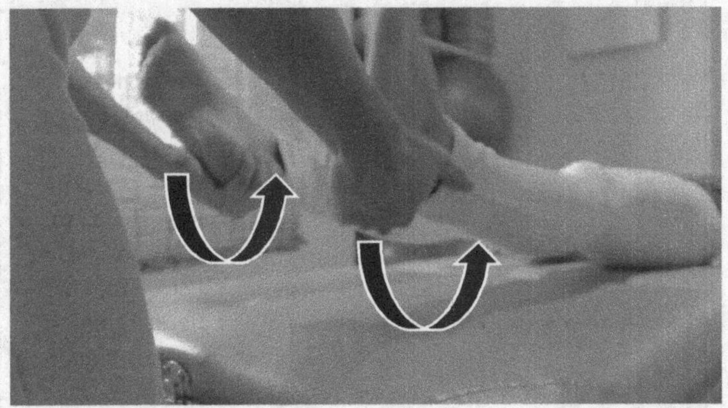

9. Then grasp the feet from the heels, and shake them. You can also rotate and pull the legs (the pull may decompress the hip joint). Note that these techniques are easier to apply on the table, as they place less strain on the therapist's lower back (especially if he or she is treating a heavy client).

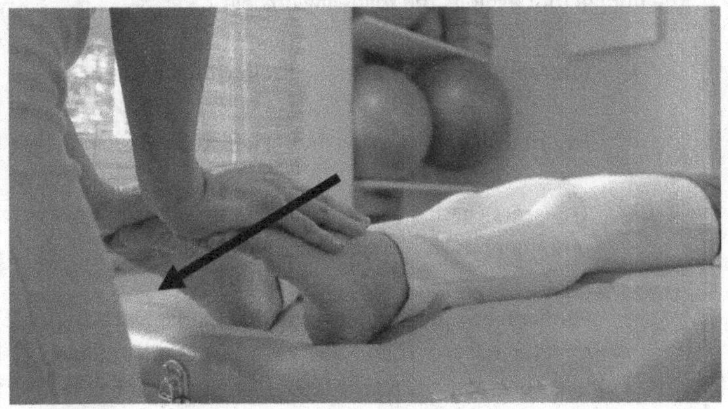

10. Conclude the session with a light stretch on the feet.

Arches of the foot

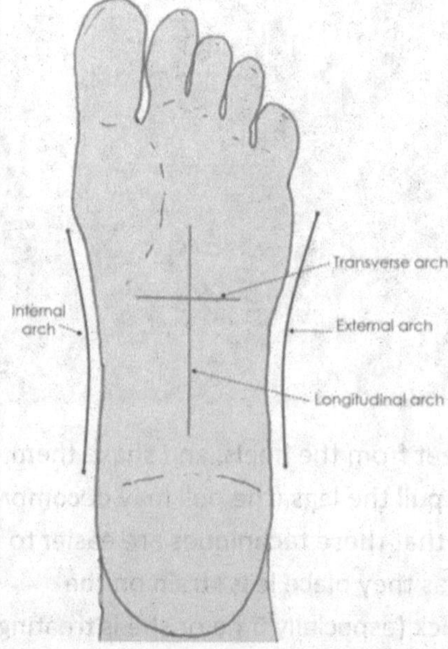

The arches of the foot are formed by the layout of the bones of the foot. Thanks to these arches, the human foot is flexible and possesses many capacities when we walk or stand.

The human foot exhibits the following arches:

- Internal arch. Also called medial longitudinal arch.

- External arch. Also called lateral longitudinal arch.

- Transverse arch. In a healthy foot, this arch is not as prominent as the fundamental longitudinal arch.

- Fundamental longitudinal arch. The fundamental longitudinal arch is contributed to by both the medial longitudinal arch and the lateral longitudinal arch. It is the large arch in the middle of the foot.

Bones of the foot

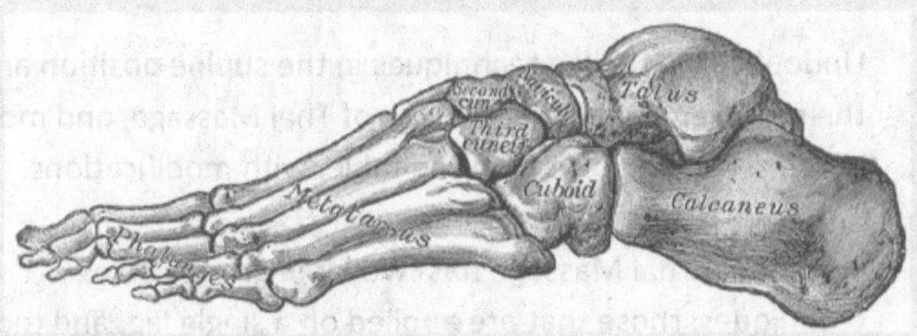

The human foot has more bones that any other part of the body. It contains 28 bones, 33 joints and about 100 small ligaments. Thanks to this complex structure, the human foot is flexible and able to perform a great variety of movements, and is able to absorb the impact of movement.

The foot can be subdivided into the forefoot, the midfoot, and the hindfoot.

The forefoot is composed of 14 phalanges, which compose the toes (the big toe contains two phalanges, while the rest contain three), as well as of five proximal long bones forming the metatarsus.
The midfoot is composed of five irregular bones: the cuboid, navicular, and three cuneiform bones.
The hindfoot is composed of the talus (or ankle bone) and the calcaneus (or heel bone). The two long bones of the lower leg, the tibia and fibula, are connected to the top of the talus to form the ankle.
The tarsus is composed of seven bones: the cuboid, navicular, and three cuneiform bones, the talus and calcaneus (that is, of the midfoot and the hindfoot).

Other important anatomical elements include the subtalar and the ankle joint. The movements produced at this joint are dorsiflexion and plantaflexion of the foot, while the subtalar joint allows inversion and eversion of the foot. These two joints connect the foot with the two long bones of the lower leg, the tibia and fibula.

The legs

Undoubtedly, the leg techniques in the supine position are the most representative feature of Thai Massage, and most of them can be applied on the table, with modifications.

Traditional Thai Massage has two large groups of leg techniques: those that are applied on a single leg, and those that involve both legs at the same time. In Thai Table Massage, we are able to apply most of the techniques of the first group, but it is difficult to apply the techniques that involve both legs.

Of course, it is possible to do all the Sen work on the legs. Actually, it is much more comfortable for the therapist to do this work on the table.

Some of these techniques are gentle and may be applied even to the elderly. However, some of them are unsuitable for older clients. Some techniques should never be applied to those who suffer from osteoarthritis of the hip.

If applied properly, these techniques can be effective not only for disorders of the legs, but also for lower back pain and sciatica. During their application, the therapist should respect the receiver's flexibility and boundaries. Clearly, you should never push the body beyond its limits.

The experienced therapist may use various props (pillows, yoga bricks, etc.), in order to support properly the receiver's body. This may be necessary especially if the receiver is an elderly person, a person with limited mobility or simply a person with limited flexibility.

Techniques for the legs

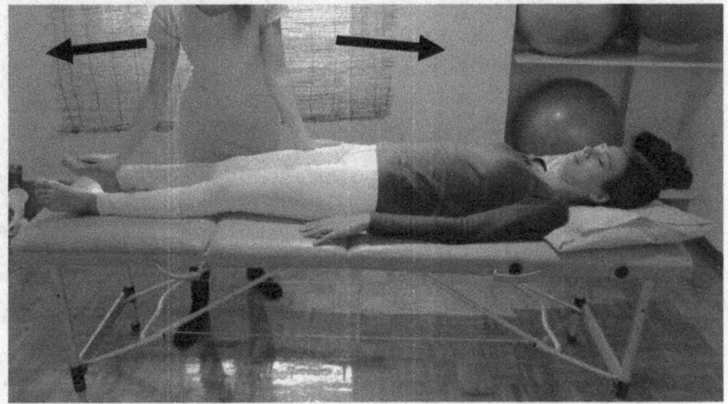

11. Start from the 3 outer lines. First stretch the meridians, by placing one palm on the receiver's ankle, and one palm on the quadriceps muscle. Breathe in. When you breathe out, use your body weight in order to apply the stretch.

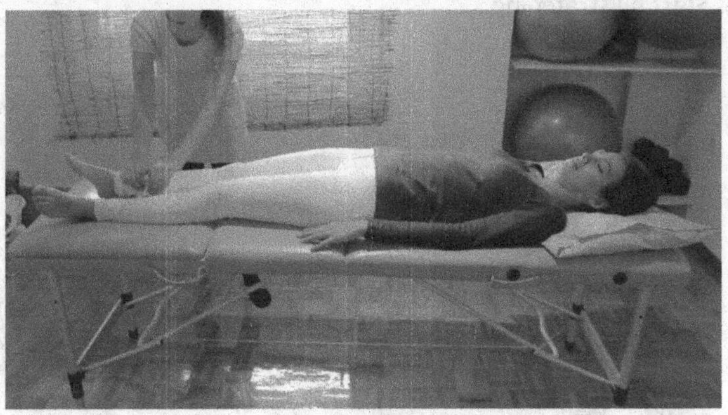

12. Then walk with your palms on the outer lines (Sahatsarangsi & Tawaree, and Itha & Pingkala). This is supposed to "warm" the meridians. Skip the knee.

Then, using your thumbs, press the 3 outer Sen. Work from the feet towards the hips, and then return. Then repeat the warming (palm walking), and the stretch.

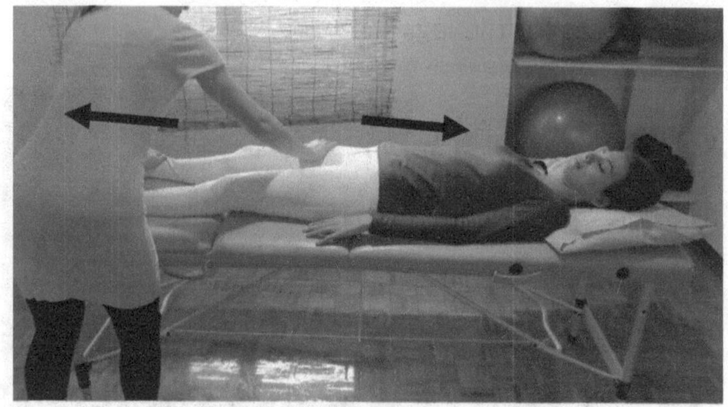

13. Then work on the Sen lines of the inner leg (these are Sahatsarangsi & Tawaree, and Kalatharee). From the supine position, it is possible to work only on the two inner lines, as the Itha & Pingkala posterior branch runs on the back of the legs and is inaccessible from the supine position.

Start by stretching…

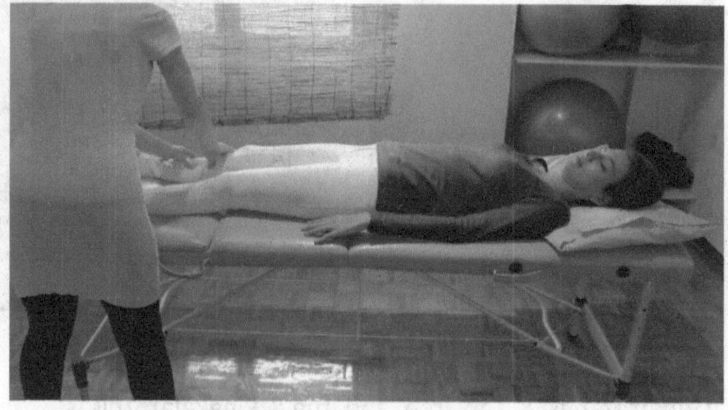

14. Then do palm walking and thumb walking. Conclude the Sen work by repeating the palm walking and the stretch.

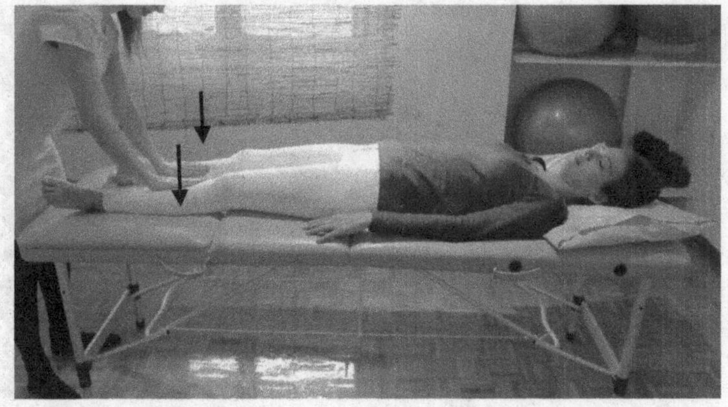

15. Using your hypothenar eminence, walk with your palms on the inner side of the lower leg. Do alternative presses and work slowly. Begin above the ankle and proceed towards the knees.

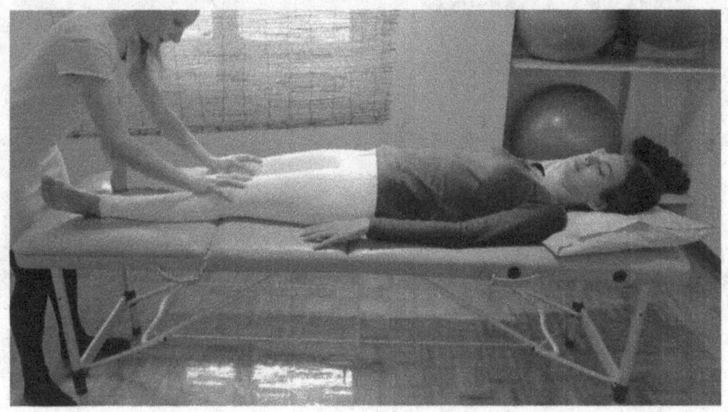

16. When you reach the knees, grasp them both and rotate the knee joint gently.

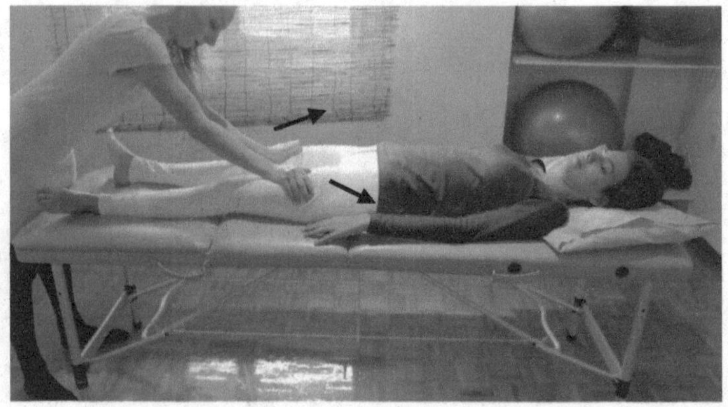

17. Then continue walking on the thighs with your palms. Do alternative presses and work slowly. Return on the receiver's feet, by repeating the previous techniques in a reverse way (that is, apply Step 16 and then Step 15).

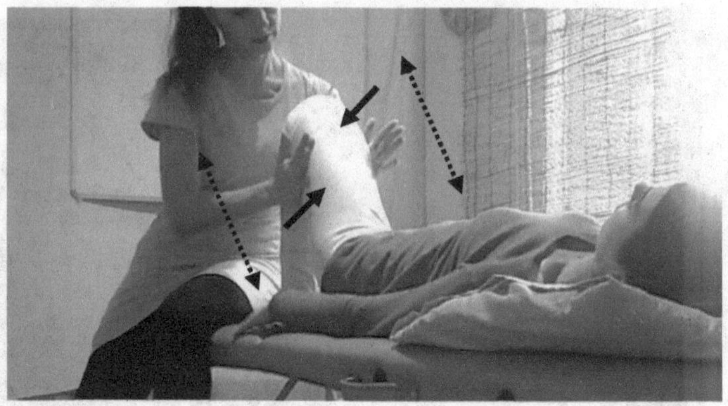

18. Lock the leg of the receiver by sitting on his or her foot with your thigh. Do a warm up on the thigh with your palms, moving upwards and downwards. Cover the entire thigh, as this technique is a sort of warm-up for the next steps. Repeat 5-10 times, depending on how tight the muscles are.

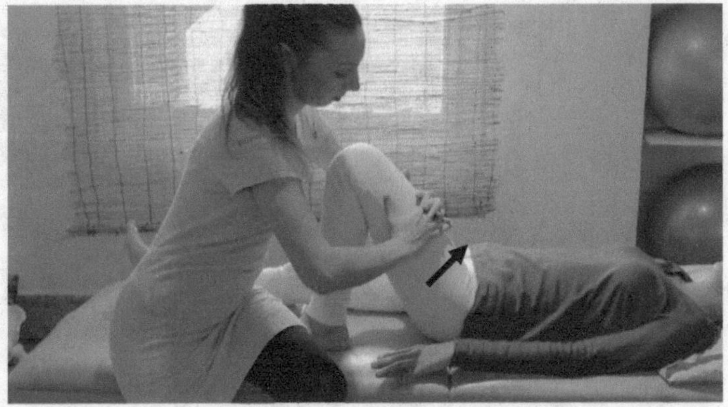

19. Still at the previous lock, interlock your fingers and try to "separate" the quadriceps muscle from the surrounding tissues. You should actually try to lift the quadriceps muscle, not to squeeze it.

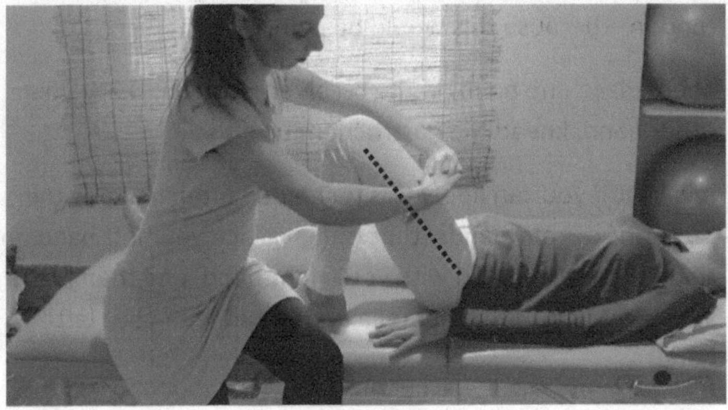

20. Then, interlock your fingers as shown in the photo, and using your thumbs, apply pressure on the 1st inner and 1st outer Sen lines.

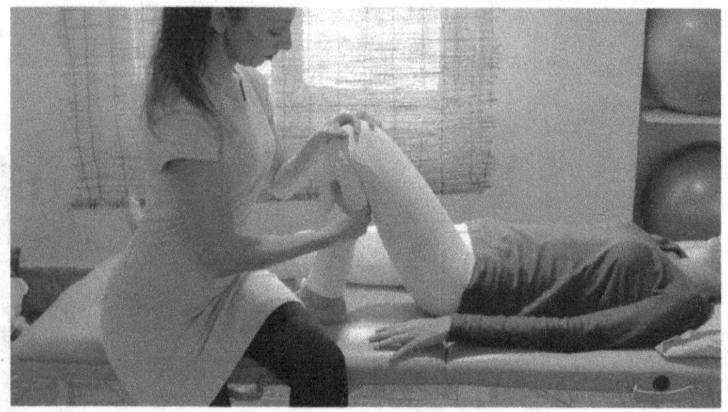

21. Stabilize the receiver's lower leg between your thighs. Using your fingers, try to separate the heads of the gastrocnemius muscle. Be careful not to continue this technique below the muscle – that is, on the Achilles tendon – because this would be painful.

Then, place one palm on the receiver's patella. Using your other hand, knead the gastrocnemius muscle.

It is best if you can apply this technique interchanging the positions of your hands (that is, first place your left hand on the patella and knead with your right hand, and then place your right hand on the patella and knead with your left hand).

This is actually the best position for work on the gastrocnemius muscle, because the therapist can access the entire muscle.

Pelvic tilt

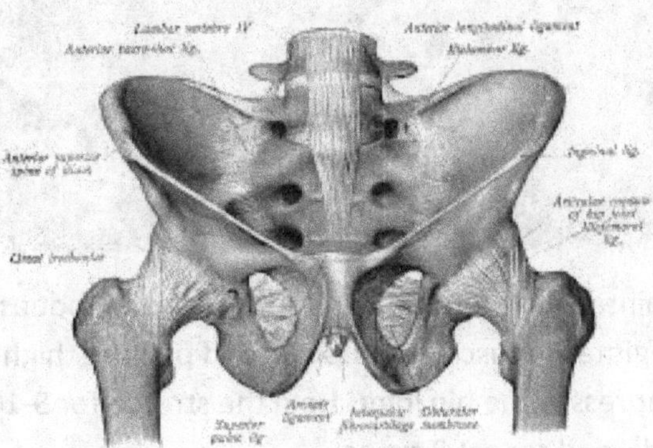

Pelvic tilt is the orientation of the pelvis in respect to the thighbones and the rest of the body. The pelvis can tilt towards the front, back, or either side of the body.

Anterior pelvic tilt (also known as lumbar lordosis) is when the front of the pelvis drops in relationship to the back of the pelvis. For example, this happens when the hip flexors shorten and the hip extensors lengthen. It can cause a height loss of 0.5-2.5 inches.

Posterior pelvic tilt is the opposite, when the front of the pelvis rises and the back of the pelvis drops. For example, this happens when the hip flexors lengthen and the hip extensors shorten, particularly the gluteus maximus which is the primary extensor of the hip.

Lateral pelvic tilt describes tilting toward either right or left and is associated with scoliosis or people who have legs of different length.

Anterior pelvic tilt and posterior pelvic tilt are very common abnormalities in regard to the orientation of the pelvis. Thai Massage, thanks to its stretches, can help to balance an abnormal pelvic tilt. Exercise is also important.

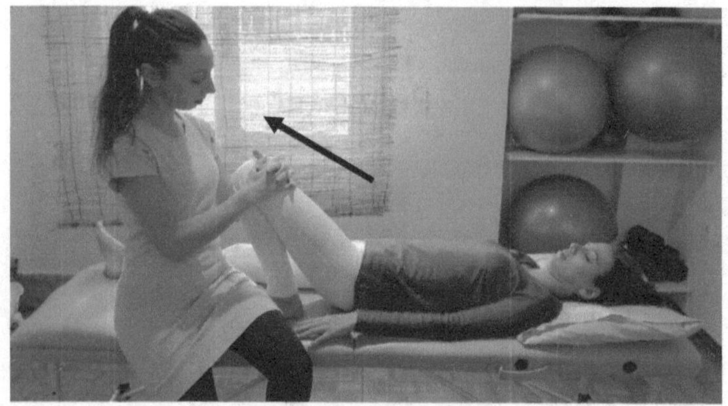

22. Maintaining the lock, bring the receiver's foot as close to her gluteus muscle as possible, and pull the thigh – this decompresses the hip joint. Hold the stretch for 5-10 seconds, and repeat 3 times.

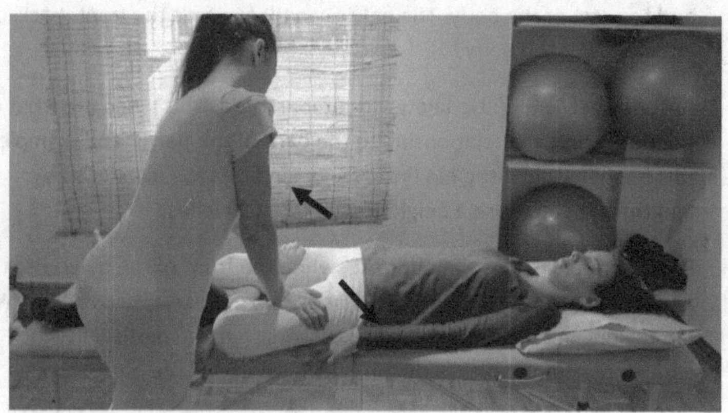

23. Release the previous leg lock. Bend the receiver's foot and stabilize it with your knee. The transverse arch of the receiver's foot should face her knee joint.

Then start walking with your palms on the receiver's thighs. Press the thighs alternatively. Do not apply pressure close to the knee joint.

Always go very gently with this technique, and observe carefully the receiver's facial expressions. Never go beyond the limits in this one, and whenever you apply it, be sure that you have warmed the muscles properly with the previous techniques.

This technique has some similarities with Patrick's test. Thus, any pain elicited during its application, may suggest hip joint disorders and / or sacroiliac joint dysfunction.

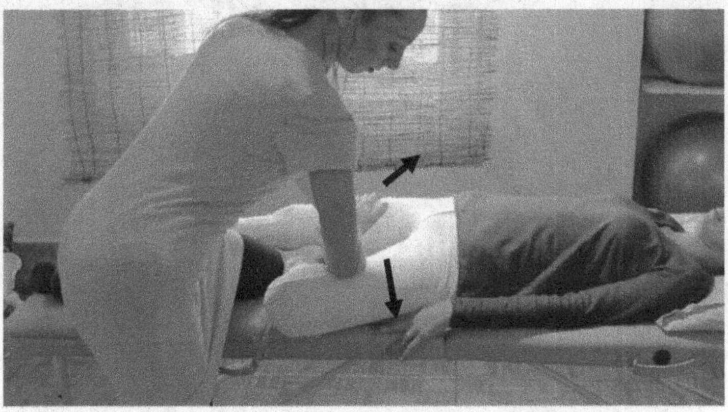

24. In this lock, you can also apply pressure with your forearm, for greater intensity. Place the hand of your other arm on the inner leg, for resistance. Steps 23 & 24 are corrective techniques for the pelvis, and they are indicated for abnormal pelvic tilt (anterior, posterior or lateral).

This and the previous technique, are contraindicated in people with hip osteoarthritis.

The hip joint

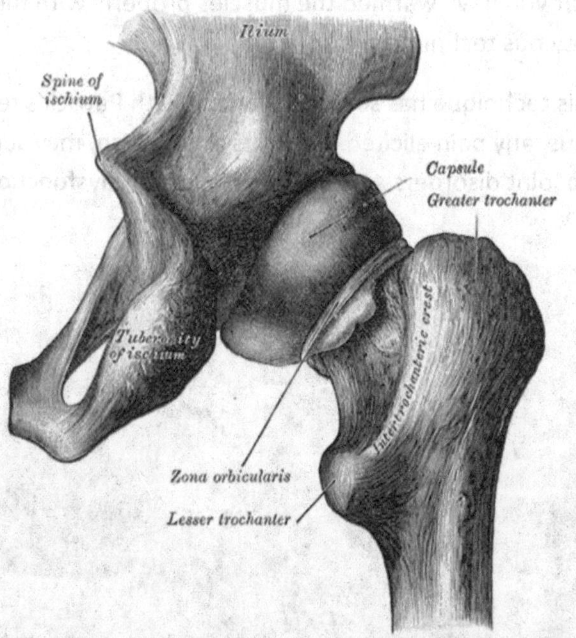

The hip joint, scientifically referred to as the acetabulofemoral joint, is the joint between the femur and acetabulum of the pelvis and its primary function is to support the weight of the body in both static (e.g. standing) and dynamic (e.g. walking or running) postures. The hip joints have very important roles in retaining balance, and for maintaining the pelvic inclination angle.

The hip joint is a synovial joint formed by the articulation of the rounded head of the femur and the cup-like acetabulum of the pelvis. It forms the primary connection between the bones of the lower limb and the axial skeleton of the trunk and pelvis. Both joint surfaces are covered with a strong but lubricated layer called articular hyaline cartilage.
Hip pain can have multiple sources and can also be associated with lower back pain.

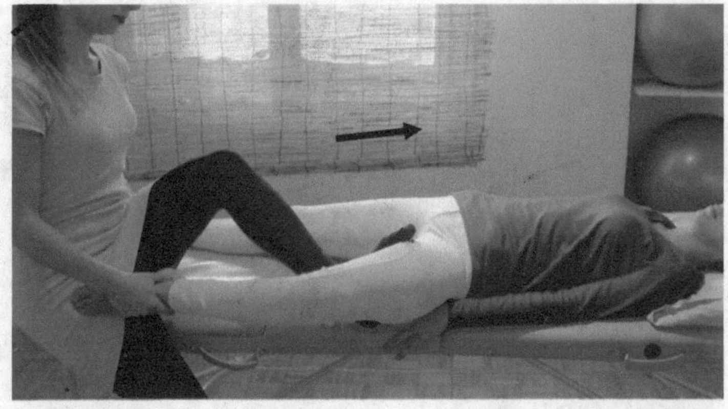

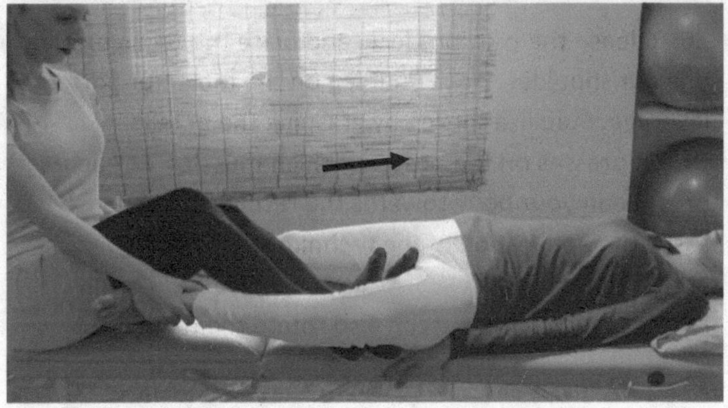

25. Grasp the receiver's ankle joints at both legs, and press the adductors with your foot. Do not pull the foot joint – just maintain a moderate resistance with your grip.

You can also sit on the massage table, and press the feet alternatively, as in the traditional Thai Massage technique on the floor.

Pressure should be applied with the transverse arch of the foot.

Do not push the thigh above the level of the hip joint, even if the receiver is flexible.

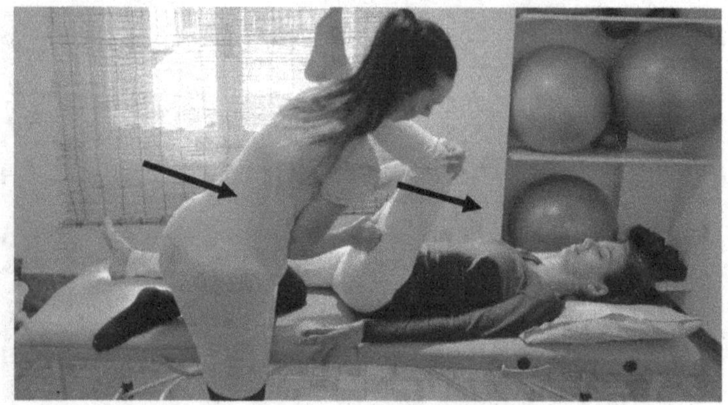

26. Release the previous lock, and place the receiver's leg on your shoulder. Place your leg on the table, for better leverage. Stabilize the leg by grasping the patella.
Do fist presses on the posterior thigh muscles. At each press, lean your body towards the receiver, in order to assist the application of the technique with your bodyweight.
From this position, you can also rotate the thigh.

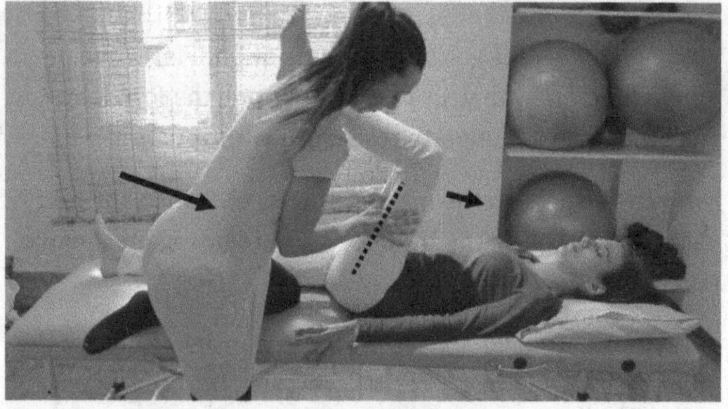

27. Same as previous step, but this is thumb pressing on the 3rd inner line (Itha & Pingkala Sen), at its posterior branch.

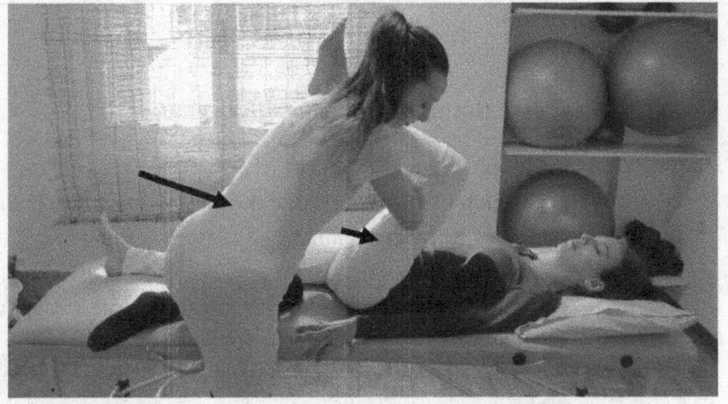

28. Same as steps 27 & 26, but in this modification I do forearm presses. My other hand is placed on the inner surface of the spread leg, for greater resistance.

This particular technique stretches the psoas muscle in the spread leg, and the gluteus and piriformis muscles of the bent leg. It is the most intense from these three techniques that actually target all the muscles of the hip.

Have in mind that muscle groups are not isolated systems. Hips muscles form an integrated system with muscles of the spine, shoulder, neck, core, and lower leg, in order to adjust our position and stability.

Thus, you should include this techniques in a session for neck pain, and even explain this fact to the receiver, who may wonder why you are doing this kind of work since he came to you complaining of tension in the shoulder or neck area.

The muscles of the hip

The muscles of the hip consist of four main groups.

- Gluteal group
  The gluteal muscles include the gluteus maximus, gluteus medius, gluteus minimus, and tensor fasciae latae.
- Adductor group
  The adductor brevis, adductor longus, adductor magnus, pectineus, and gracilis make up the adductor group.
- Iliopsoas group
  The iliacus and psoas major comprise the iliopsoas group. Together these muscles are commonly referred to as the "iliopsoas".
- Lateral rotator group
  This group consists of the externus and internus obturators, the piriformis, the superior and inferior gemelli, and the quadratus femoris.

Functions

Movements of the hip occur because multiple muscles activate at once. Most muscles are also responsible for more than one type of movement.

- The psoas is the primary hip flexor, assisted by the iliacus. The pectineus, the adductors longus, brevis, and magnus, as well as the tensor fasciae latae are also involved in flexion.
- The gluteus maximus is the main hip extensor, but the inferior portion of the adductor magnus also plays a role.
- The adductor group is responsible for hip adduction.
- Medial rotation is performed by the gluteus medius and gluteus minimus, as well as the tensor fasciae latae and assisted by the adductors brevis and longus and the superior portion of the adductor magnus.
- Each muscle of the lateral rotator group causes lateral rotation of the thigh. These muscles are aided by the gluteus maximus and the inferior portion of the adductor magnus.

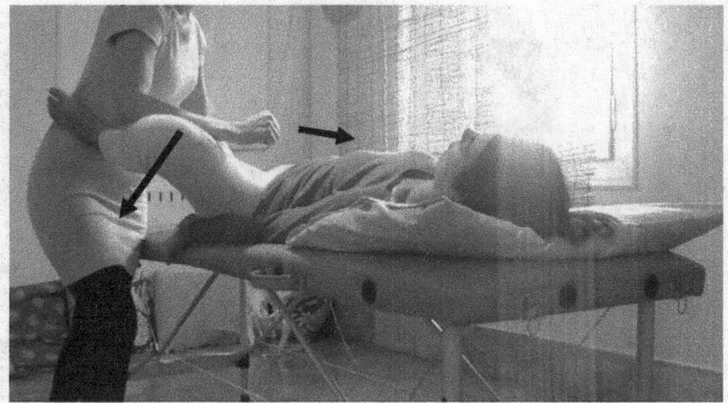

29. Place the receiver's foot above your iliac crest, and start stretching gently her adductors. One hand should be places on the receiver's bent leg, and one on the spread leg.

At each stretch, lean your body towards the receiver and bring your pelvis forward, in order to assist the application of the technique with your bodyweight.

Apply the technique very slowly and observe the body's structural limitations. Repeat 4-5 times.

I always do this technique when a client complains of lower back pain, as this occurs often because of tight adductors. Inflexible adductors are very common, especially in people with desk jobs and sedentary lifestyle.

In traditional Thai Massage on the floor, the therapist stabilizes the receiver's foot on the upper part of the quadriceps muscle. This is equally stable with the table modification, although the iliac crest forms a more definite "barrier" for the lock.

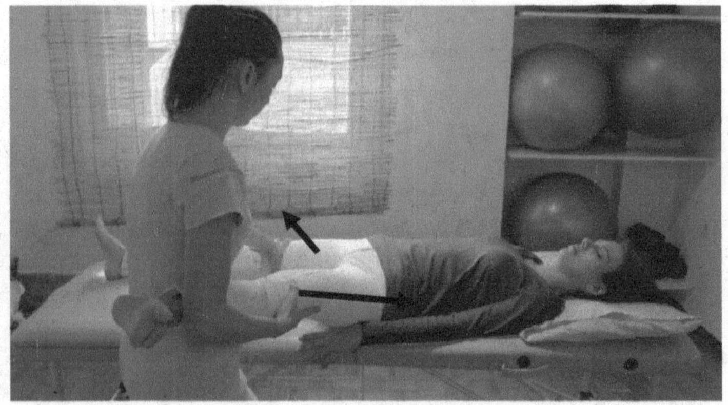

30. This technique also targets the adductor muscles. Place the receiver's lower leg above your iliac crest, and hold it with your arm. Place your other hand on the adductor muscles of the spread leg for resistance and stability of the lock. Bring the stretched leg forward very slowly, and hold the stretch 5-10 seconds each time.

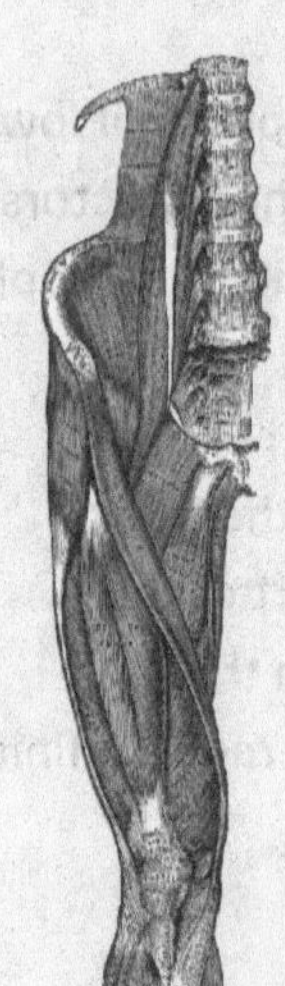

Adductor muscles of the hip

The adductors originate on the pubis and ischium bones and insert mainly on the medial posterior surface of the femur.

This muscle group consists of:

- Adductor brevis
- Adductor longus
- Adductor magnus
- Adductor minimus. This is often considered to be a part of adductor magnus.
- Pectineus
- Gracilis

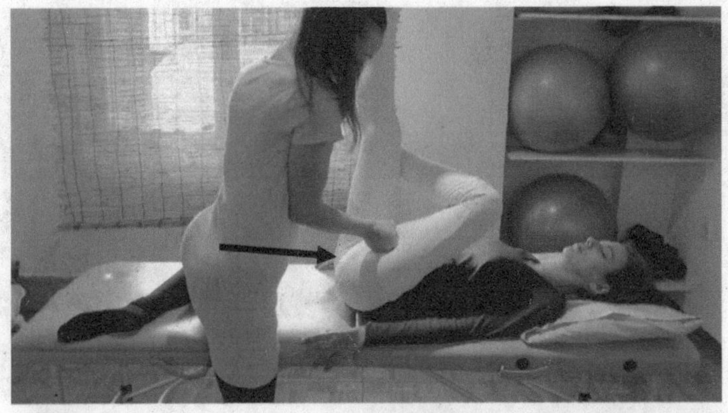

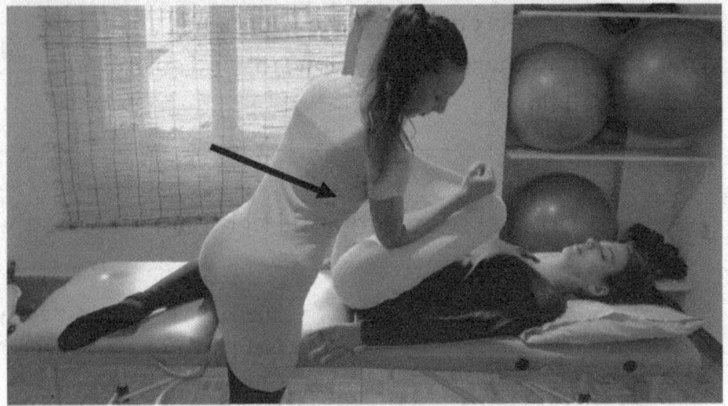

31. Place your knee on the table, and lock the receiver's lower leg above the knee joint. Her ankle should be placed outside of her thigh. Press the posterior thigh muscles with your fist, and simultaneously push the other leg towards the receiver's head.

You can also press with your forearm and elbow.

At each press, lean your body towards the receiver and bring your pelvis forward, in order to assist the application of the technique with your bodyweight.

This is a good technique for sciatica. However, do not push the legs too far if the receiver has a slipped disc.

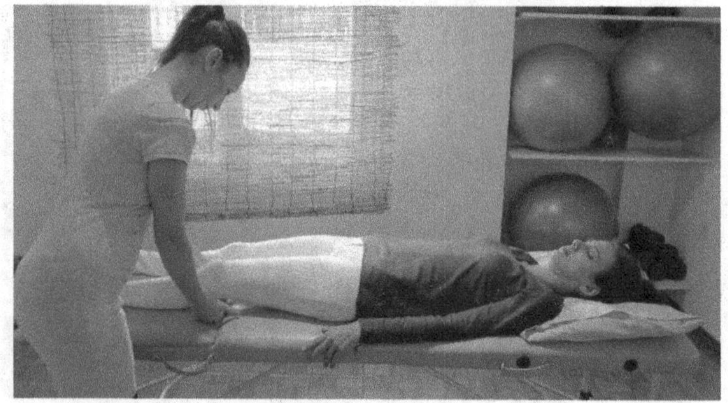

32. In order to relax the leg, place your hands under the knee joint, and shake it gently upwards and downwards. Repeat 8-10 times.

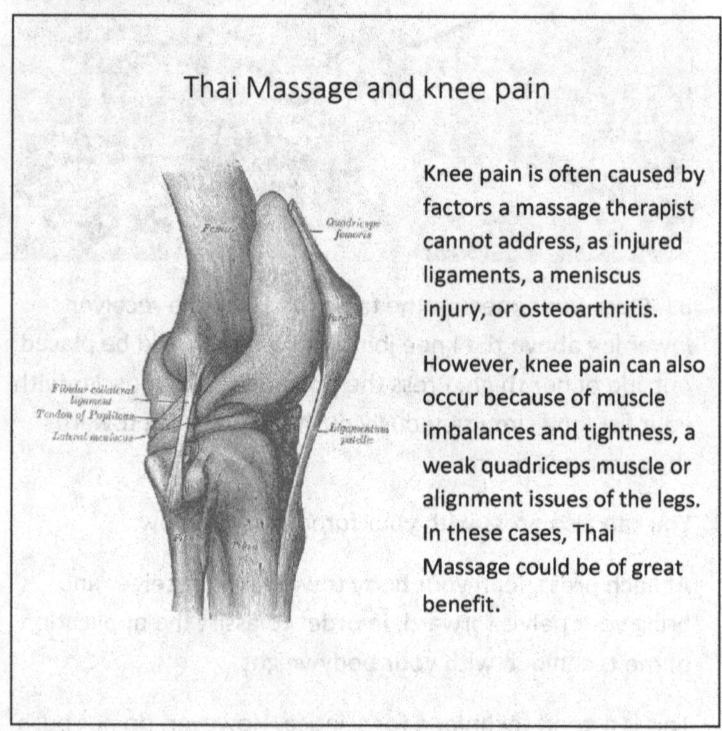

Thai Massage and knee pain

Knee pain is often caused by factors a massage therapist cannot address, as injured ligaments, a meniscus injury, or osteoarthritis.

However, knee pain can also occur because of muscle imbalances and tightness, a weak quadriceps muscle or alignment issues of the legs. In these cases, Thai Massage could be of great benefit.

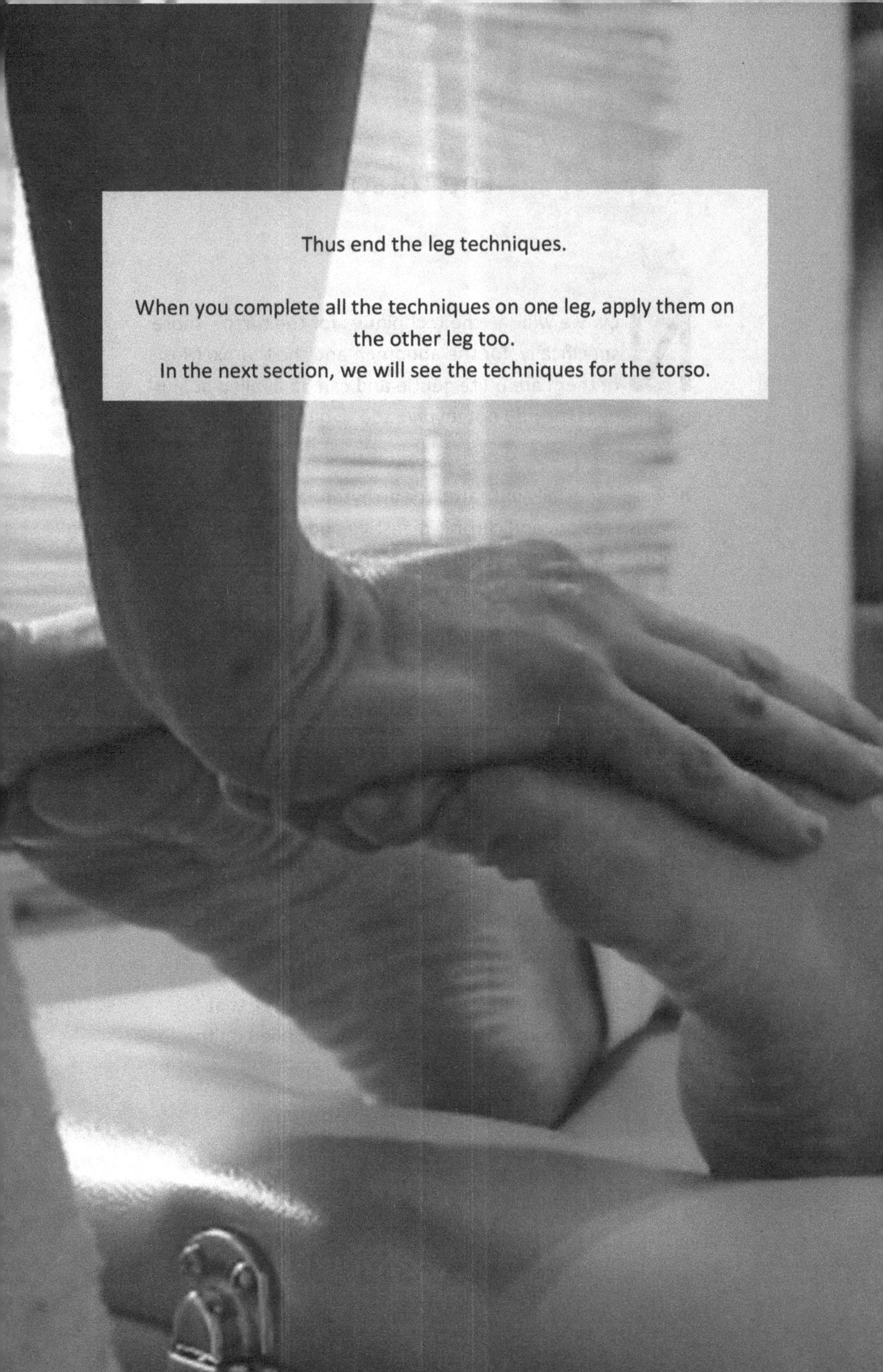

Thus end the leg techniques.

When you complete all the techniques on one leg, apply them on the other leg too.
In the next section, we will see the techniques for the torso.

The torso

Now we will see the techniques for the torso – more specifically, for the abdomen and the thorax. Most of them are quite gentle and can be applied at any age group, as they do not involve too dynamic mobilizations.

They are especially indicated for arrhythmias, stress, nervous tension, and chronic digestive and breathing disorders. Moreover, some abdominal techniques can also be helpful for lower back pain.

If you intend to work for some time on the trunk, please place a pillow under the receiver's knees. This will help proper pelvis alignment.

The following techniques (especially the techniques for the thorax) are more effective when combined with hot herbal packs.

It is more comfortable for the therapist, to perform these on the table than on the floor. For the techniques of the abdominal cavity, feel free to sit on a stool, as none of them requires you to lean and use your bodyweight.

Those trained in traditional Thai Massage will see that I included some techniques that cannot be applied on the floor.

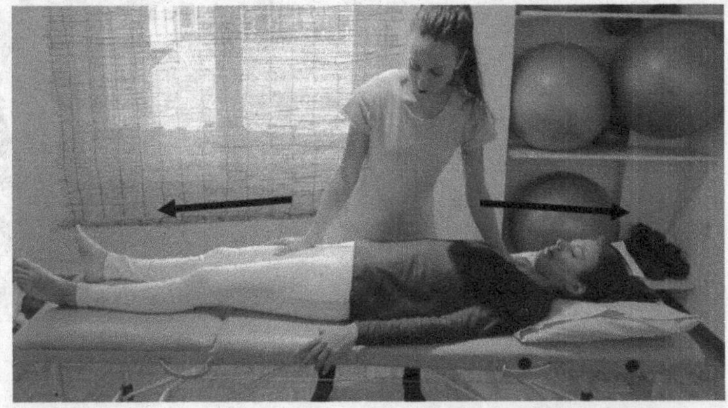

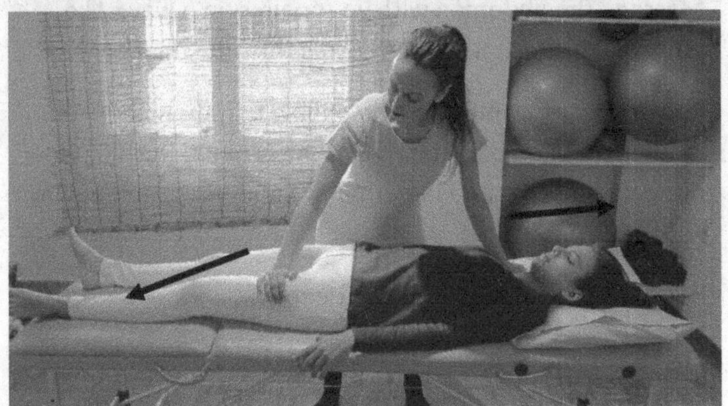

33. Do four stretches on the torso. Place one palm on the receiver's shoulder, and one palm on the quadriceps muscle. Apply two stretches with your palms on the same side of the receiver's body, and two stretches with your palms on opposite sides. It does not matter from which stretch or from which side you will start.

This is an excellent technique. Not only it "opens" the torso, preparing the area for deeper work, but it is also helpful for lower back pain, as it decompresses slightly the lumbar spine. It is also indicated for lateral pelvic tilts.

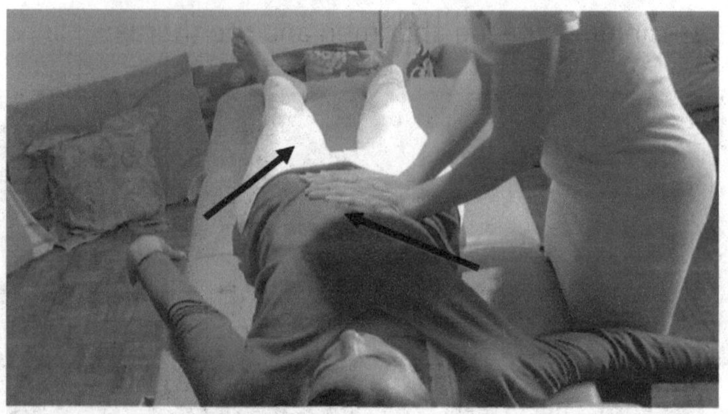

34. I like to call this technique the "wave".

Massage the abdomen with your palms, in a wave-like pattern. This technique stimulates the intestinal peristalsis.

You are basically pushing and pulling the abdomen. Your movement should be parallel to the ground. Pushing is done with thenar and hypothenar eminences, and pulling with your fingers.

Repeat 5-10 times, slowly and deeply.

This technique is indicated for lower back pain, constipation, dysmenorrhea, and breathing problems. It should never be applied if there are enlarged organs in the area (spleen or liver), and in cases of menorrhagia.

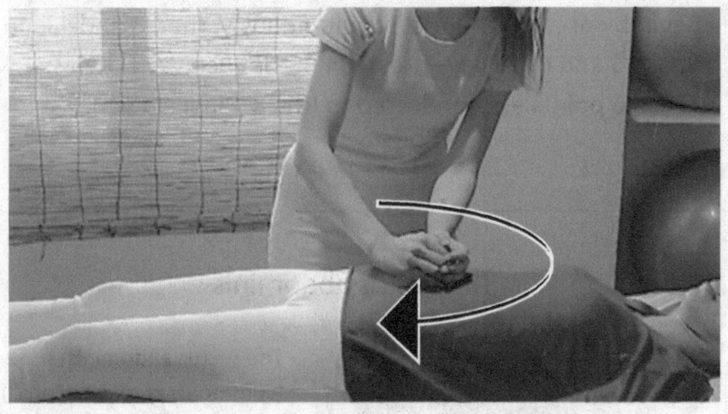

35. I like to call this technique the "cup".
Place your palms on the abdomen, and rotate the
hypothenar eminence slowly around the umbilicus. Use
your body weight – do not apply direct pressure with your
hands. Work clockwise.

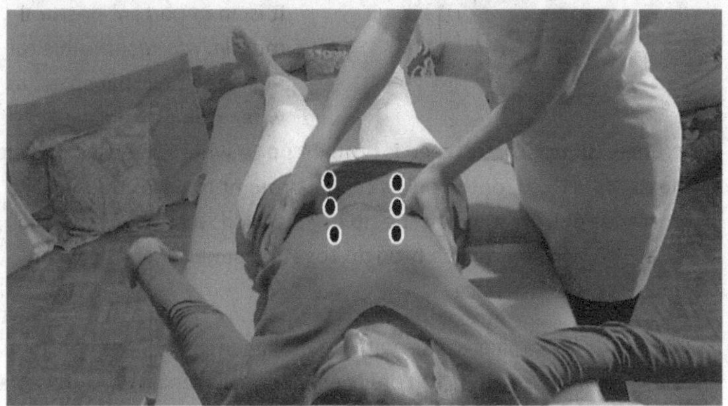

36. Now press 6 points next to the rectus abdominis
muscle.

Points 1 and 2 are located two fingers beside the umbilicus,
and two fingers above its level. Points 3 and 4 are also
located two fingers beside the umbilicus, and at the same
level with it. Points 5 and 6 are located two fingers beside
the umbilicus, and two fingers below its level.

Begin by pressing 1 and 2 simultaneously, then 3 and 4, and finally 5 and 6. Always press when the receiver exhales. These 6 points are connected to Itha & Pingkala Sen.

The rectus abdominis

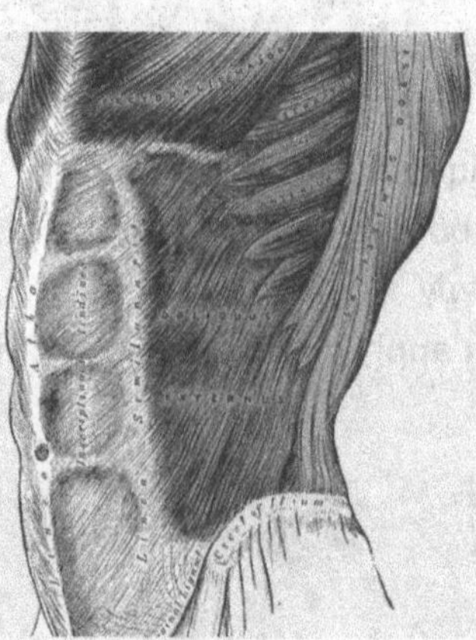

The rectus abdominis (commonly known as "abs") is a long flat muscle, which extends along the whole length of the front of the abdomen, and is separated from its fellow of the opposite side by the linea alba.

It is an important postural muscle. It is responsible for flexing the lumbar spine, as when doing a so-called "crunch" sit up. The rib cage is brought up to where the pelvis is when the pelvis is fixed, or the pelvis can be brought towards the rib cage (posterior pelvic tilt) when the rib cage is fixed, such as in a leg-hip raise. The two can also be brought together simultaneously when neither is fixed in space.

The rectus abdominis assists with breathing and plays an important role in respiration when forcefully exhaling, as seen after exercise as well as in conditions where exhalation is difficult such as emphysema. It also helps in keeping the internal organs intact and in creating intra-abdominal pressure, such as when exercising or lifting heavy weights, during forceful defecation or childbirth.

Its poor coordination or tightness, may contribute to chronic low back pain. Moreover, some types of back pain can be caused by rectus abdominis trigger points.

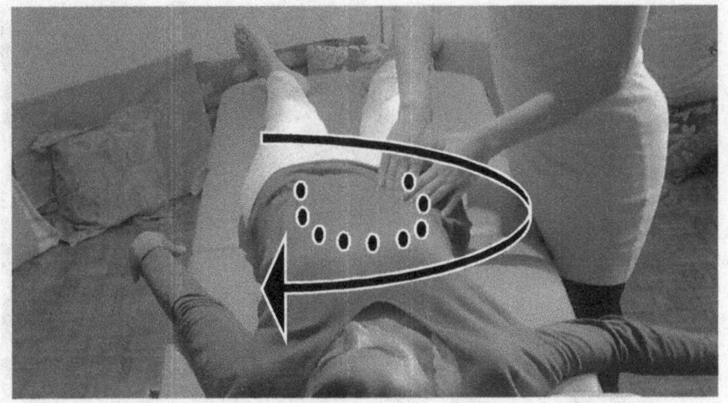

37. Press 9 points around the umbilicus, in a clockwise direction.

Points 1 and 9 are located above the superior anterior iliac spine, while 5 is located below the xiphoid process. The other points are distributed evenly on this "circle", on the belly.

The 9 Points are connected to Nantakawat Sen. However, as Point 5 is specifically connected to Sumana Sen, it is used for breathing disorders, and problems pertaining to the heart and the mind. It is located on the diaphragm.

The diaphragm

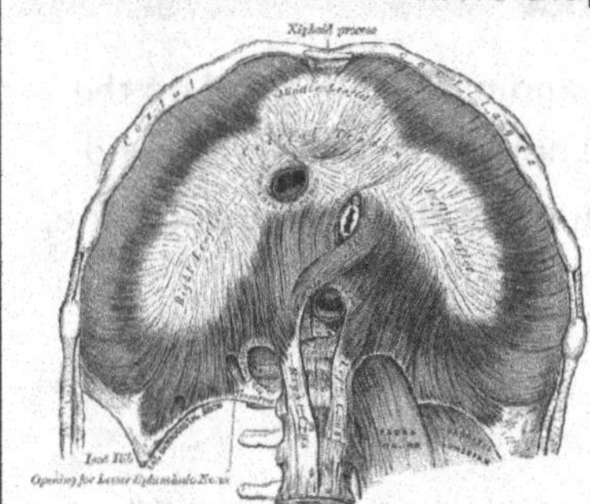

The diaphragm is a sheet of internal skeletal muscle. It separates the thoracic cavity from the abdominal cavity, and it is the main muscle of respiration.
It has a powerful connection to our emotions.

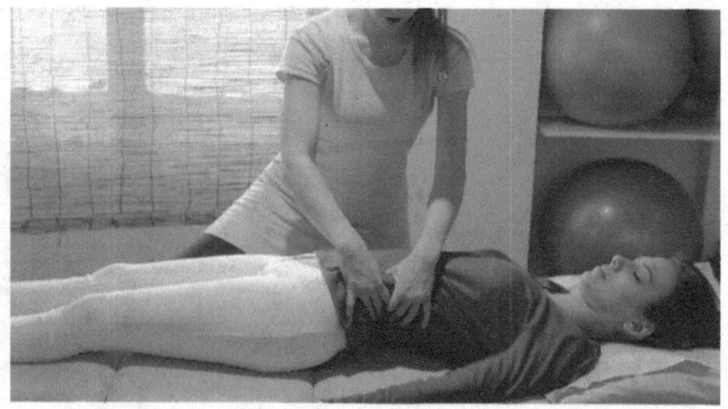

38. Do some kneading on the lateral side of the torso, above the pelvis. Excellent technique for lower back pain.

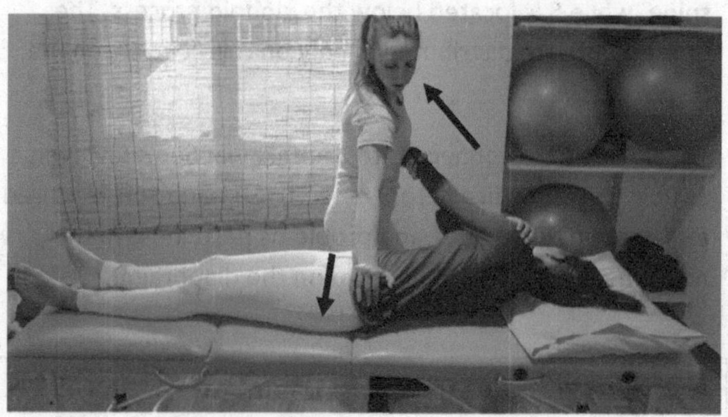

39. Grasp the receiver's arm, and place your hand on the iliac crest. Pull the arm, while holding the iliac crest, and rotate the torso. This technique targets the thoracic spine.

Repeat 3 times, at both sides of the torso.

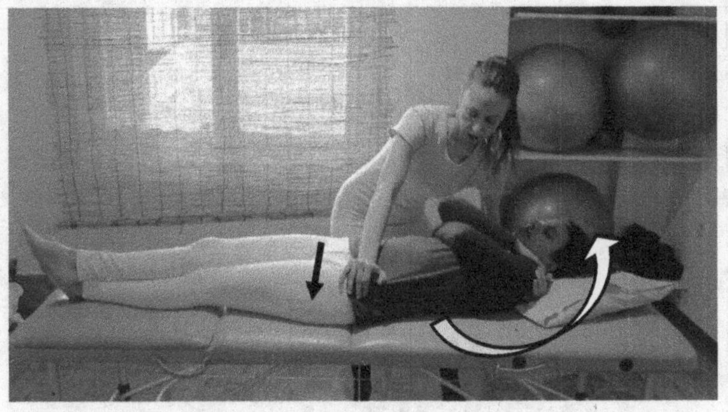

40. I like to call this technique "the banana"!

Have the patient cross her arms, and cross her legs. Place your hand on the iliac crest, and slide your other arm under the receiver's locked arms. Pull the client's torso. This technique stretches the quadratus lumborum, a deep muscle that is related to lower back pain.

Repeat this technique 3 times at both sides of the torso, and hold the stretch at least for 10 seconds each time. You will find that each time you perform it, the receiver will have a better range of motion than the previous time.

This is a "must" technique for lower back pain. Since it does not involve any disc compression, it can be applied safely to any patient with degenerative disc disease.

The quadratus lumborum

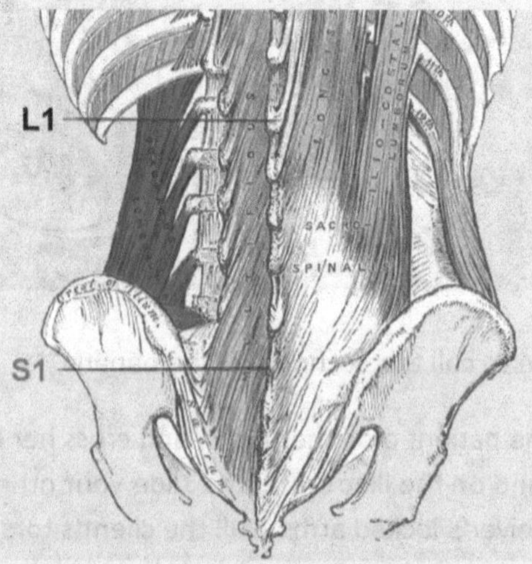

Because the QL connects the pelvis to the spine and is therefore capable of extending the lower back when contracting bilaterally, the two QLs pick up the slack, as it were, when the lower fibers of the erector spinae are weak or inhibited (as they often are in the case of habitual seated computer use and/or the use of a lower back support in a chair).

Given their comparable mechanical disadvantage, constant contraction while seated can overuse the QLs, resulting in muscle fatigue. A constantly contracted QL, like any other muscle, will experience decreased blood flow, and, in time, adhesions in the muscle and fascia may develop, the end point of which is muscle spasm.

This chain of events can be and often is accelerated by kyphosis, which is invariably accompanied by rounded shoulders, both of which place greater stress on the QLs by shifting body weight forward, forcing the erector spinae, QLs, multifidi, and especially the levator scapulae to work harder in both seated and standing positions to maintain an erect torso and neck.

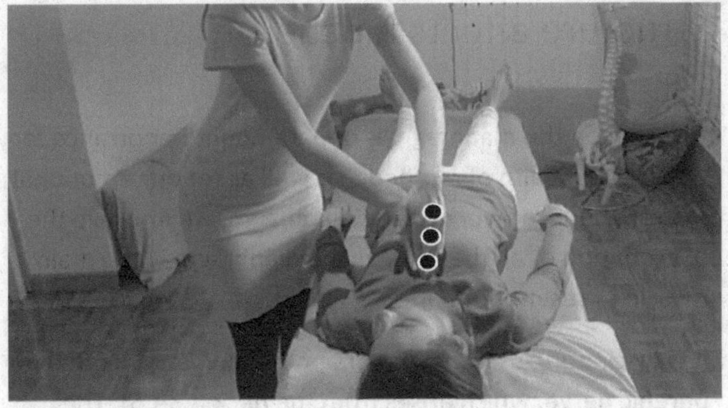

41. Rub softly three points on the sternum, with your index and middle fingers. These points are indicated for stress and breathing problems.
It is best if you combine these techniques with hot herbal packs. Be sure to add eucalyptus, peppermint and camphor, as these herbs are expectorant and calming for the mind.

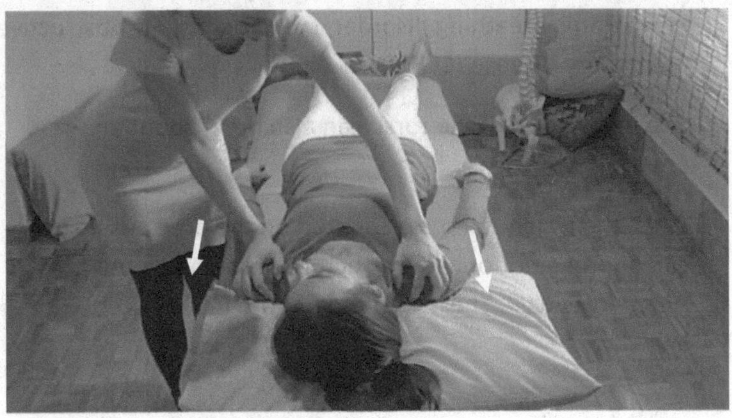

42. Press softly the shoulders, as the receiver exhales.
This concludes the techniques for the torso.

Structure affects function

Working on the diaphragm is of paramount importance for the overall health of our body, as well as for our emotional state. Whenever work on the diaphragm, we improve the oxygenation of all the cells, as the diaphragm is the main muscle of respiration.

It is fascinating that the diaphragm is innervated by the phrenic nerve, which arises from the neck (C3-C5). The phrenic nerve also controls breath - if both phrenic nerves are severed, life is terminated. Moreover, the diaphragm, from an embryological point of view, originated from the neck, from a structure (septum transversum) that unfolds in a downward direction during gestation.

The Thai acupressure points of technique 37, especially those that are located on the diaphragm, can be used for any chronic breathing disorder, even for chronic obstructive pulmonary disease (COPD).

The techniques of the torso can also bring about an emotional release.

Thus, the mobilizations presented on the previous pages, can improve not only the structure of the body, but its function as well. These two aspects are interrelated anyway.

Arms and Hands

Arm and hand techniques are generally gentle, and can be applied almost to all age groups. They are indicated especially for neck pain (numbness in the arms originates from the neck, as these areas are connected neurologically), stress, shoulder pain, and of course pain localized on the arm and the hand. They work especially well when combined with warm herbal packs and heat rubs.

The Kalatharee Sen arm branch has a definite connection to the heart, at an energetic level. Thus, work on this sen can be beneficial for arrhythmias – especially if they are due to stress.

Work on the Itha & Pingkala Sen branches of the arms and hands is indicated for tendonitis and overuse disorders.

The therapist should be careful not to apply dynamic arm stretches to clients who have had shoulder dislocation and / or have loose shoulder ligaments or general instability of this area.

All the techniques should be applied to both arms and hands.

Techniques for the arm and the hand

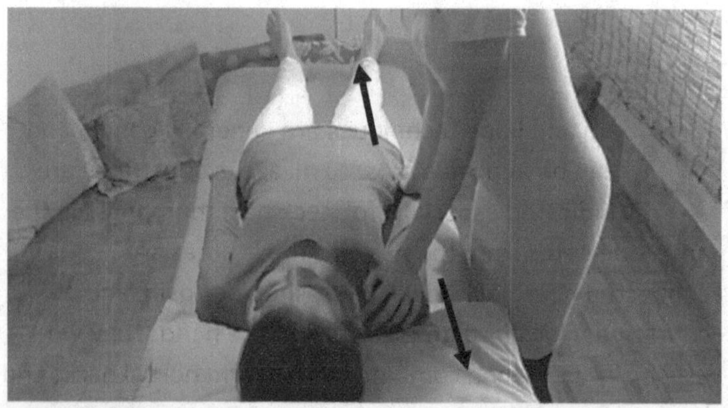

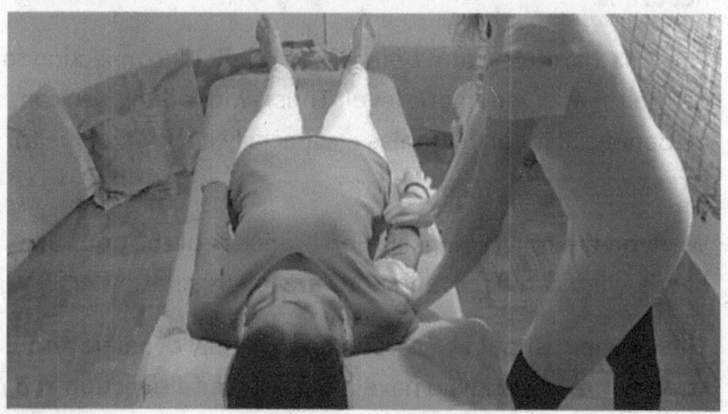

43. Work on the arm Sen lines. Start with Itha & Pingkala Sen, and do all the 5 steps of Jap Sen.

Then turn the arm and work on the inner surface, on the Kalatharee Sen line. Again, do all the 5 steps of Jap Sen.

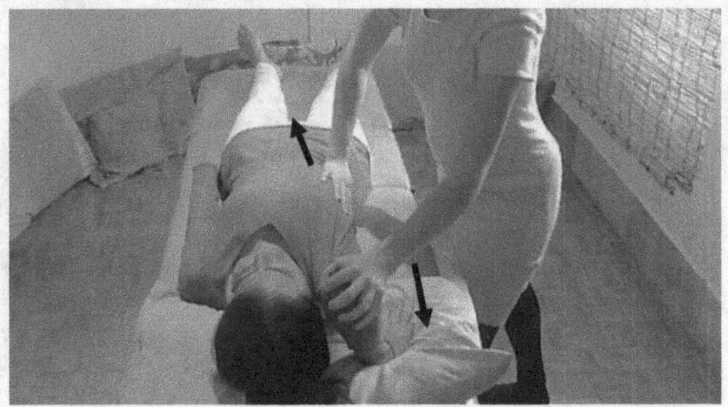

44. Place the arm in the "triangle" position: Ask the receiver to bend her arm, with her fingers pointing to her shoulder. Holding firmly the arm from the elbow, grasp and pull the ribs, creating space in the thoracic cage. Recommended for postural kyphosis and breathing problems.

The rib cage

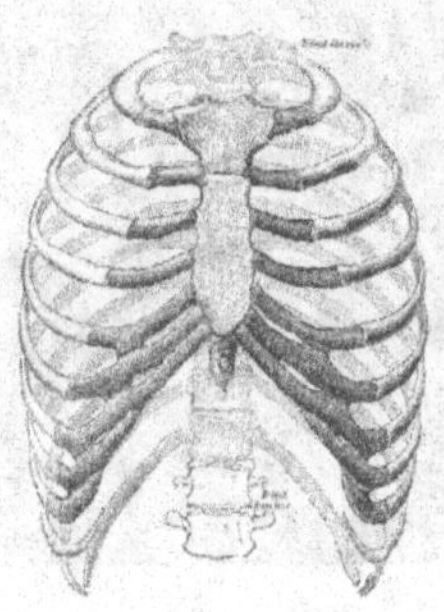

The first seven sets of ribs, known as "true ribs", are attached to the sternum by the costal cartilages. The first rib is unique and harder to distinguish than other ribs. It is a short, flat, C-shaped bone. The vertebral attachment can be found just below the neck at the first thoracic vertebra, and the majority of this bone can be found above the level of the clavicle.

Ribs 2 through 7 have a more traditional appearance and become longer and less curved as they progress downwards. The following five sets are known as "false ribs", three of these sharing a common cartilaginous connection to the sternum, while the last two (11th and 12th ribs) are termed floating ribs. They are attached to the vertebrae only, and not to the sternum or cartilage coming off of the sternum.

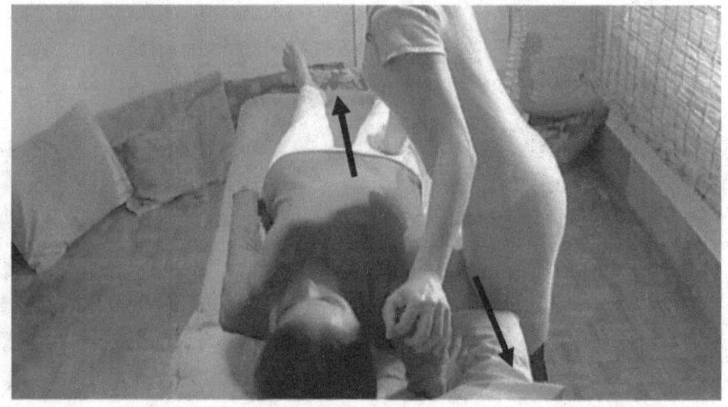

45. Maintaining the "triangle" lock, place one hand on the receiver's quadriceps muscle, and one arm on the elbow. Stretch the torso. Repeat three times.
Recommended for lateral pelvic tilt.

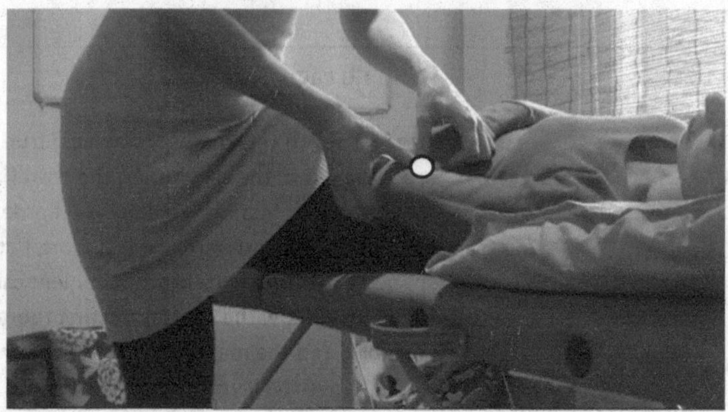

46. Place your thigh on the table, and rest the receiver's arm on it. Do Thai acupressure around the elbow joint. With the elbow flexed, the point is on the lateral end of the transverse cubital crease. Heat rub is recommended, in cases of tennis elbow.

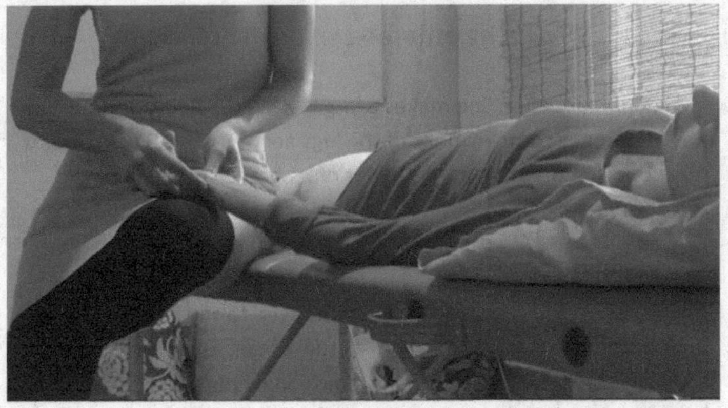

47. Sit on the table, and place the receiver's palm on your thigh. Place your little fingers next to the receiver's thumb and little finger, in order to "lock" the palm. Then, you can rub the 6 points, as shown in the illustration.

You can also massage the palm, and do a light stretch on the palmar fascia, by stretching down the receiver's little fingers. Doing this stretch while elevating the forearm, is a technique recommended for carpal tunnel syndrome and tendonitis.

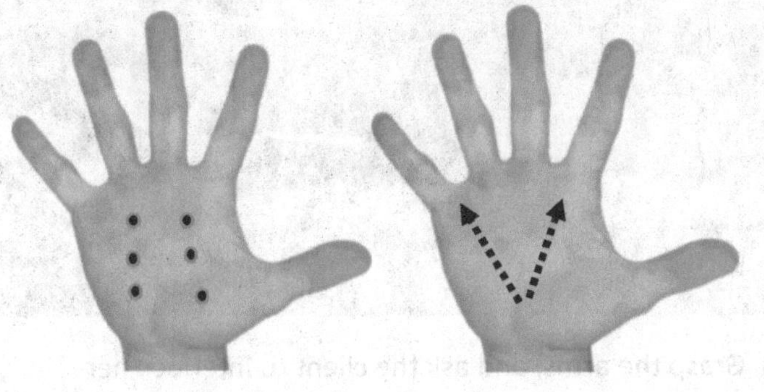

Whenever there is an issue with the elbow, or even with the shoulder or the neck, I recommend massaging the palm and the wrists with sliding massage movements.

The Kalatheree Sen palm branch

Kalatharee Sen line makes a large "X" in the body, and runs on the inner compartment of the legs and the arms. I have found out that pressing the five lines of its branch on the palm, is very relaxing.

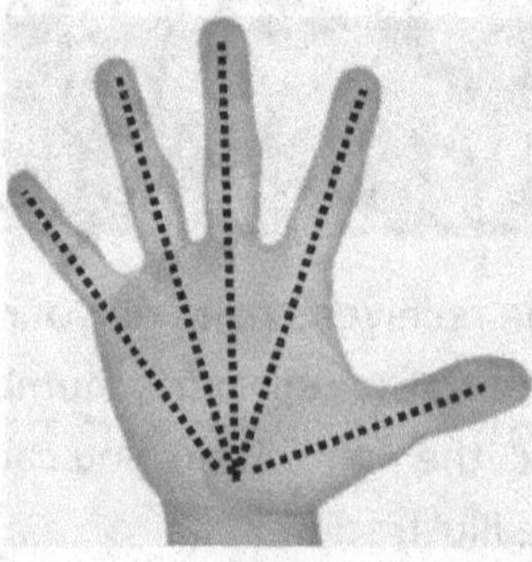

In Thai medicine, this Sen is connected to the heart (to the actual organ, as well as to the emotional heart). And, indeed, we shake hands whenever we wish to seal an agreement, as a gesture of trust, or when we want to express our love for someone. Our palms are an area we expose to someone we supposedly trust.

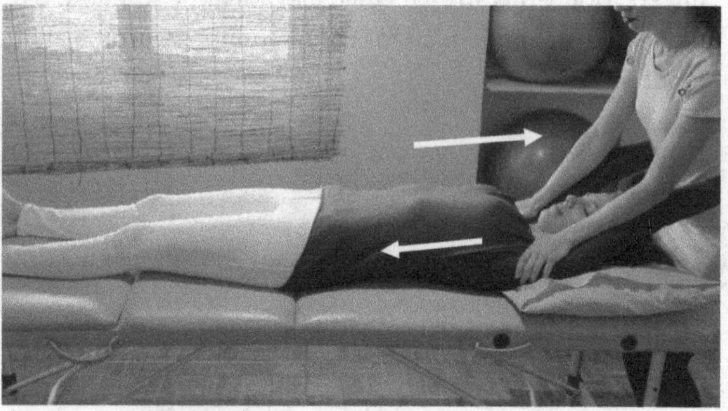

48. Grasp the arms, and ask the client to interlock her fingers behind your back. Then push her pectoralis major, while pulling your body backwards. This technique also creates space in the thoracic cage.

The shoulder joint

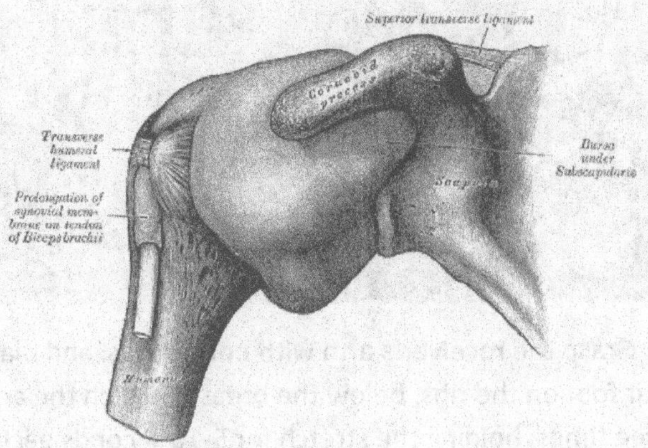

The shoulder joint is a ball and socket joint that allows the arm to rotate in a circular fashion or to hinge out and up away from the body. The joint capsule is a soft tissue envelope that encircles the glenohumeral joint and attaches to the scapula, humerus, and head of the biceps. It is lined by a thin, smooth synovial membrane. The rotator cuff is a group of four muscles that surround the shoulder joint and contribute to the shoulder's stability. The muscles of the rotator cuff are supraspinatus, subscapularis, infraspinatus, and teres minor. The cuff adheres to the glenohumeral capsule and attaches to the humeral head.

The shoulder must be mobile enough for the wide range actions of the arms and hands, but stable enough to allow for actions such as lifting, pushing, and pulling.

The muscles and joints of the shoulder allow it to move through a remarkable range of motion, making it one of the most mobile joints in the human body. The shoulder can abduct, adduct, rotate, be raised in front of and behind the torso and move through a full 360° in the sagittal plane. This tremendous range of motion also makes the shoulder extremely unstable, far more prone to dislocation and injury than other joints.

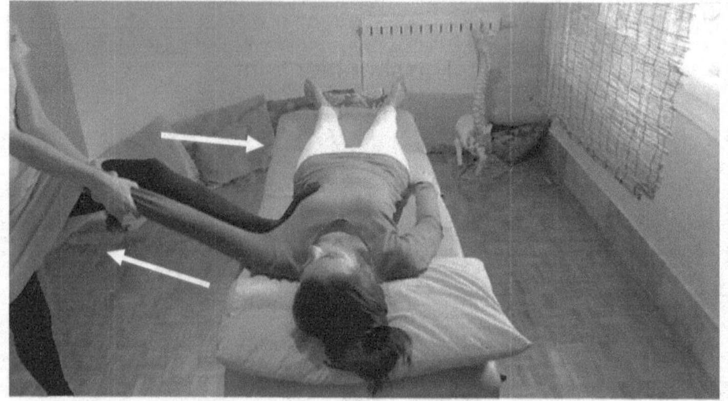

49. Grasp the receiver's arm with both hands, and place your foot on the ribs, below the breast. Stretch the arm three times, holding the stretch for 5-10 seconds each time. The technique is recommended for lateral pelvic tilts. Do not apply it on people with loose ligaments of the shoulder.

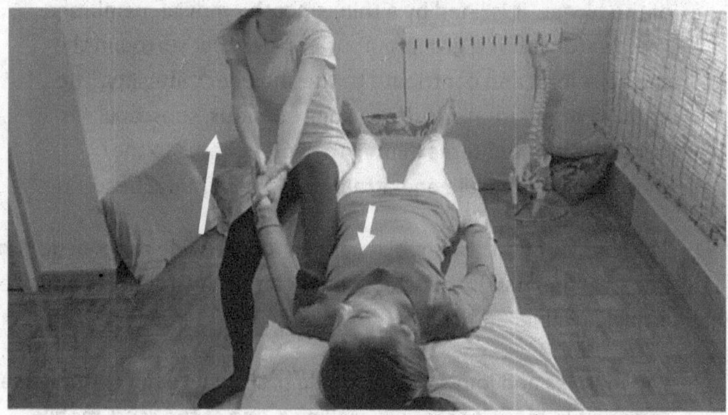

50. Sit on the table, and place your foot in the armpit. Stretch the arm – take care NOT to push your foot in the armpit.
This is a good technique for people with instability of the shoulder joint.

Side position

ow we'll see techniques for the side position. This is the most important position, as it allows us to access the whole body. If you are trained in pregnancy massage, you can perform some of these techniques on a pregnant woman as well, with the appropriate adjustments in her positioning.

Actually, a Thai Table Massage session (as well as a traditional Thai Massage session on the floor) can be comprised solely by the side position. Moreover, it is a very comfortable position for the receiver, especially for people with lower back problems, as it respects all the spinal curves.

Any technique applied to the one side of the body, should be applied on the other side too. The therapist should also be very cautious when performing back bends to clients with degenerated discs and / or spinal stenosis.

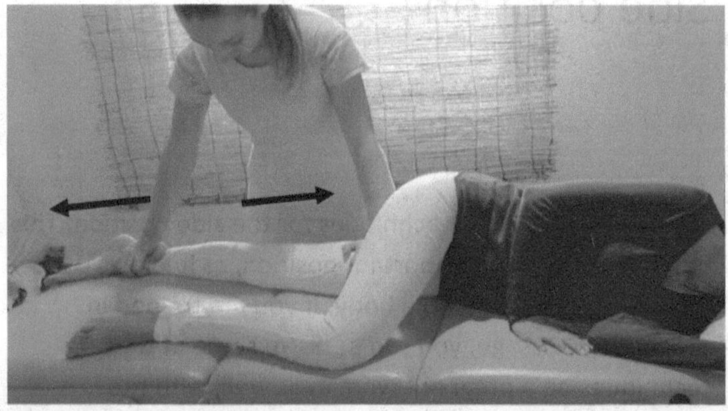

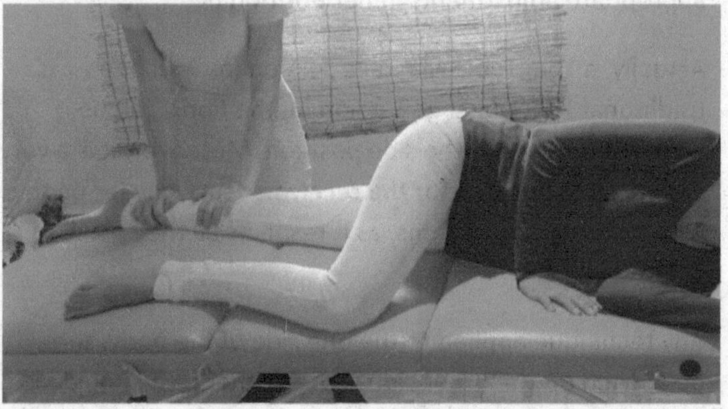

51. Start by doing Jap Sen on the lines of the inner leg. As usual, begin with stretching, and proceed with palm walking, thumb walking, again palm walking, and again stretching.

The inner leg in this position has two exposed lines: Sahatsarangsi (or Tawaree) Sen, and Kalatharee Sen. You can press them both, or just one, according to the client's needs.

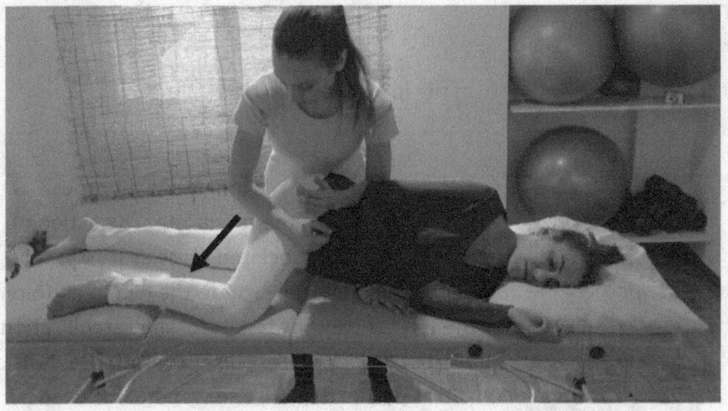

52. Place the forearm above the pelvis for resistance, and roll the forearm of your other arm on the iliotibial band (corresponds with 3rd outer line, and that's Itha & Pingkala Sen).

The forearm above the pelvis creates a light stretch on the gluteus muscles, and on the ligaments around the sacrum. When these ligaments are tense, lower back pain can occur.

A typical example of this, is tension of the iliolumbar ligament (a strong ligament passing from the tip of the transverse process of the fifth lumbar vertebra to the posterior part of the inner lip of the iliac crest).

The iliotibial band

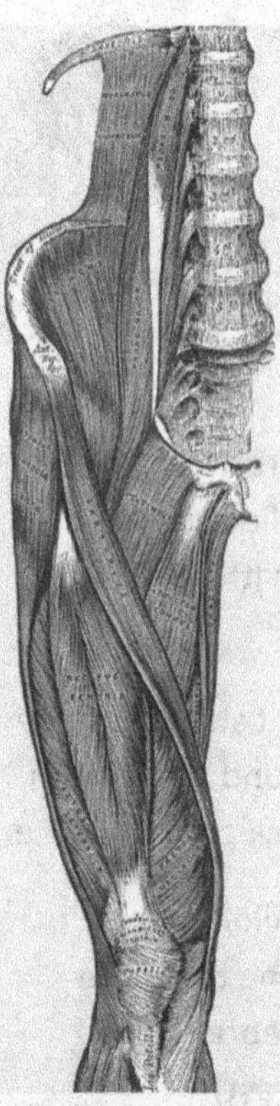

The iliotibial band is a longitudinal fibrous reinforcement of the fascia lata. The action of the ITB and its associated muscles is to extend, abduct, and laterally rotate the hip. In addition, the ITB contributes to lateral knee stabilization. The IT band stabilizes the knee both in extension and in partial flexion, and is therefore used constantly during walking and running. When a person is leaning forwards with a slightly flexed knee, the tract is the knee's main support against gravity.

The IT band is of critical importance to asymmetrical standing (pelvic slouch). The upward pull on the lower attachment of the IT band thrusts the knee back into hyperextension, thereby locking the knee and converting the limb into a rigid supportive pillar.

Iliotibial band syndrome is a common thigh injury generally associated with running, cycling or hiking. The onset of iliotibial band syndrome occurs most commonly in cases of overuse. The iliotibial band itself becomes inflamed in response to repeated compression on the outside of the knee or swelling of the fat pad between the bone and the tendon on the side of the knee. ITB syndrome can also be caused by poor physical condition.

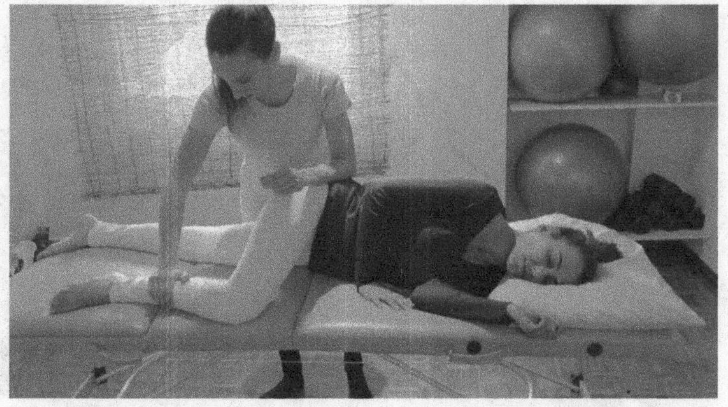

53. Do palm presses on the lower leg. Do not press the ankle.

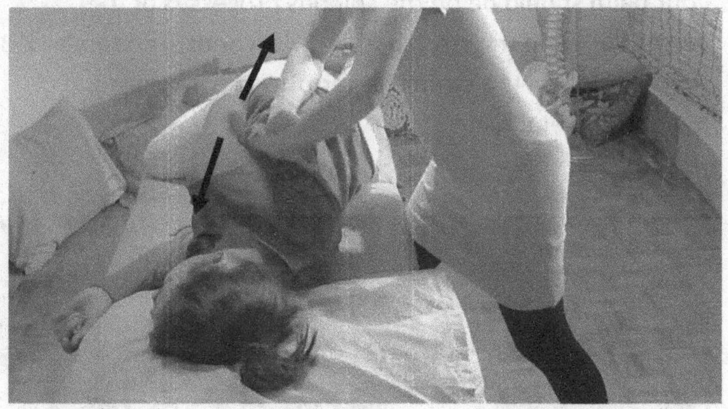

54. Place your forearm on the gluteus muscle, and create a horizontal stretch, in order to decompress the lumbar spine. Be careful not to press the elbow joint on the gluteus muscle.

It is recommended to perform a circular rubbing movement on the gluteus muscles. This technique is indicated for sciatica and lower back pain.

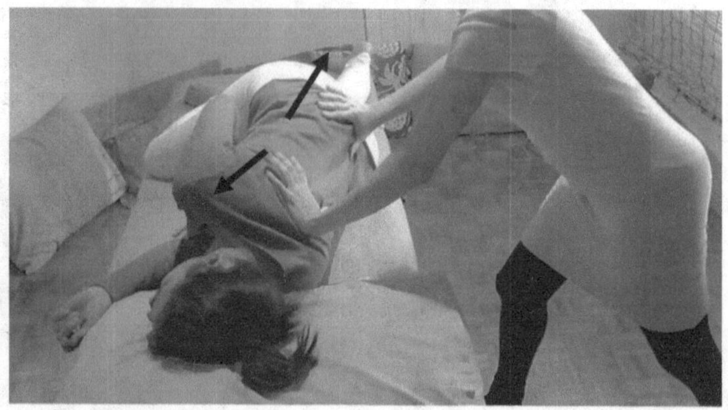

55. Place one hand on the sacrum, and one hand at the end of the thoracic spine, and stretch the back. The center of your palm should be on the spinous processes of the vertebrae. Hold the stretch for 5-10 seconds, and repeat 2-3 times. Actually, the stretch is performed with the hypothenar eminence.

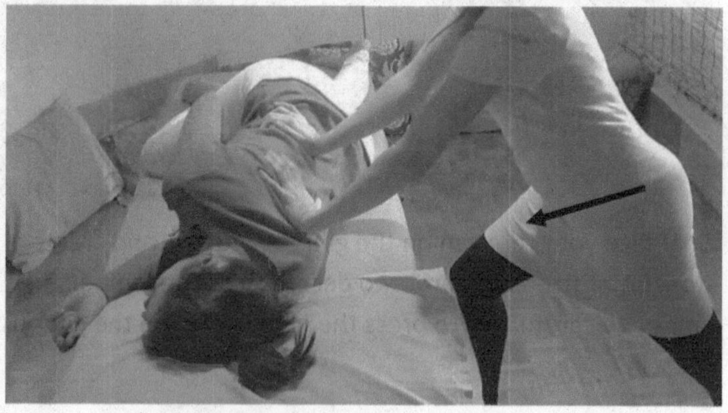

56. Do palm walking next to the spine. This is the Itha & Pingkala posterior branch. Start from the lower back, proceed towards the neck, and return to the pelvis.

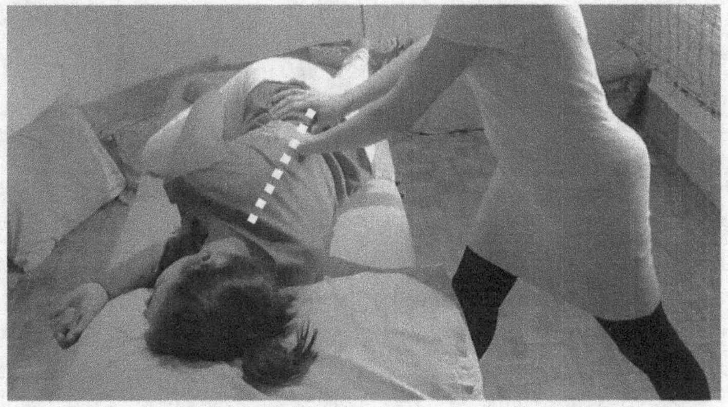

57. Then, do thumb walking on the Itha & Pingala lines, next to the spine. Start from the lower back, proceed towards the neck, and return to the pelvis.

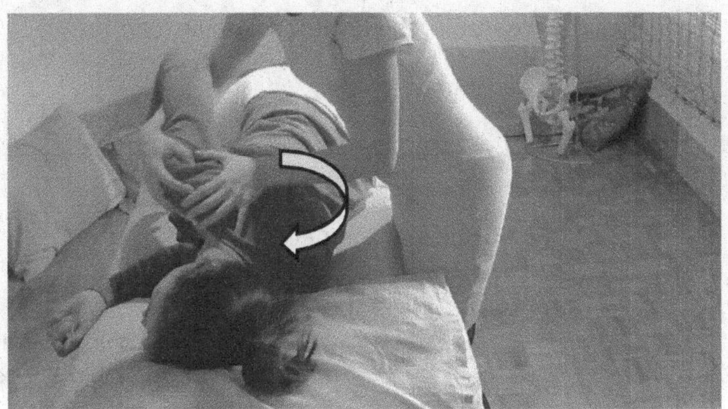

58. Grasp the receiver's shoulder and rotate it. While rotating the shoulder, you may hear cricking sounds. This may mean that the shoulder joint is unstable. In this case, you should not pull the shoulder in other techniques, especially upwards or laterally.

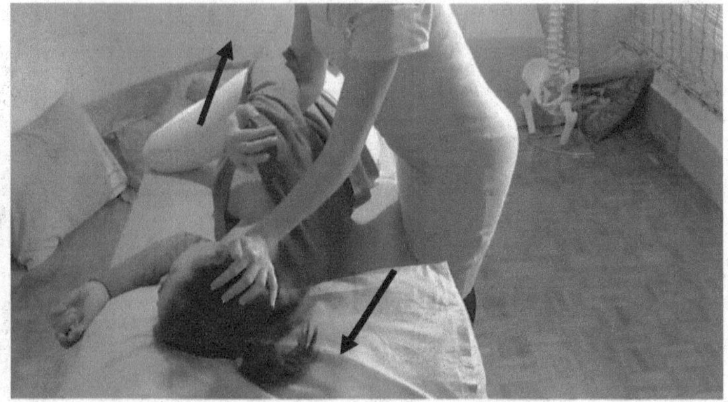

59. Place one hand on the mastoid process gently, and leave your other hand on the shoulder, as before. Pull back the receiver's shoulder, as she exhales.

Good technique for neck pain due to shortened muscles. It stretches the trapezoid, the levator scapulae, and the scalene muscles.

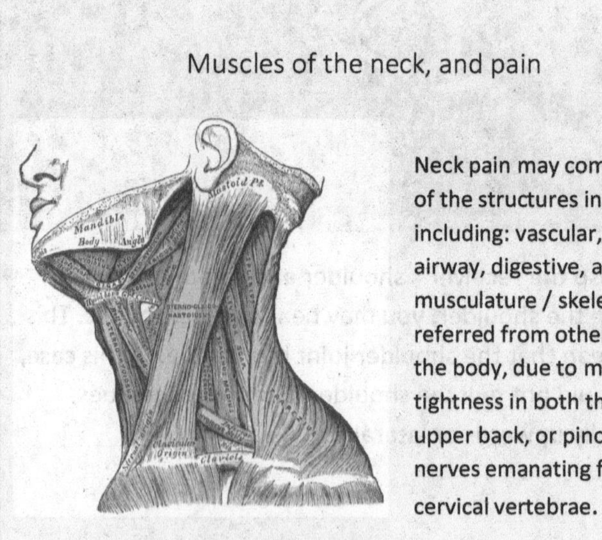

Muscles of the neck, and pain

Neck pain may come from any of the structures in the neck including: vascular, nerve, airway, digestive, and musculature / skeletal, or be referred from other areas of the body, due to muscular tightness in both the neck and upper back, or pinching of the nerves emanating from the cervical vertebrae.

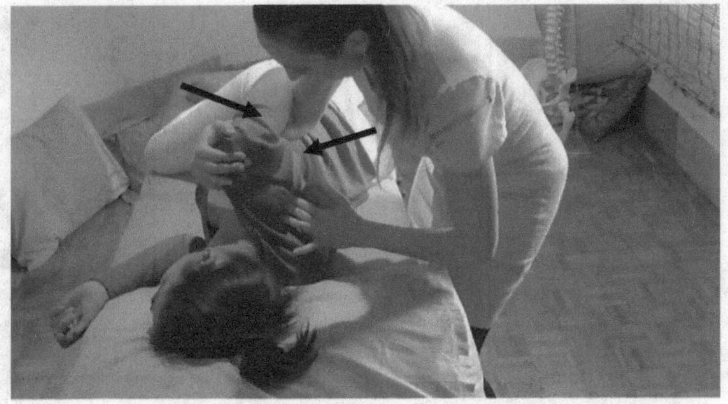

60. Place one palm in front of the receiver's clavicle, and grasp the receiver's shoulder. Insert your fingertips in the scapula, as you pull it back.

Move your fingers in many spots around the scapula, and stay 3-4 seconds on each "insertion". This technique targets the rhomboid muscles.

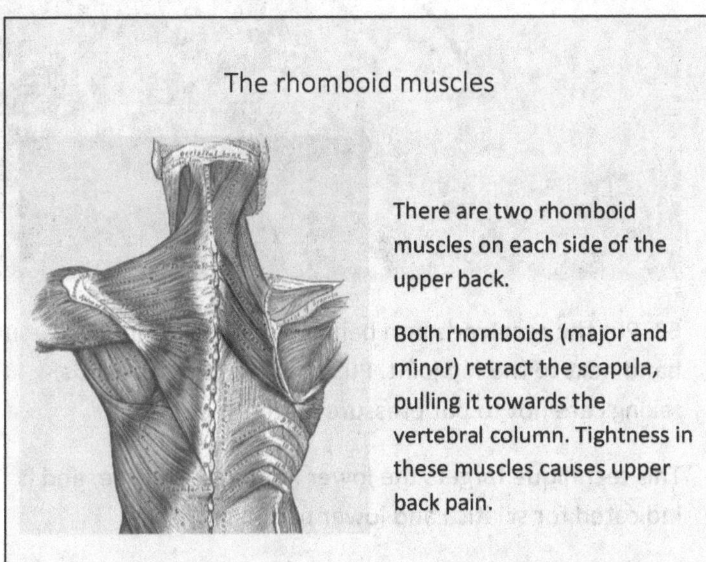

The rhomboid muscles

There are two rhomboid muscles on each side of the upper back.

Both rhomboids (major and minor) retract the scapula, pulling it towards the vertebral column. Tightness in these muscles causes upper back pain.

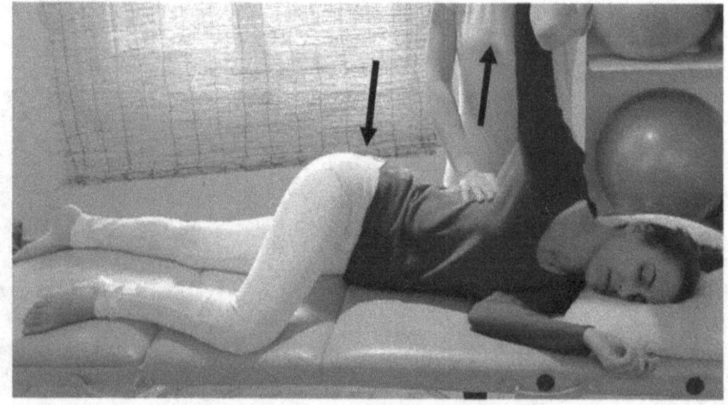

61. Raise and stretch the arm, while pressing lightly on the ribs. This technique targets the Pectoralis major muscle, and is indicated for postural kyphosis. Hold the stretch for 5-10 seconds, and repeat 3 times.

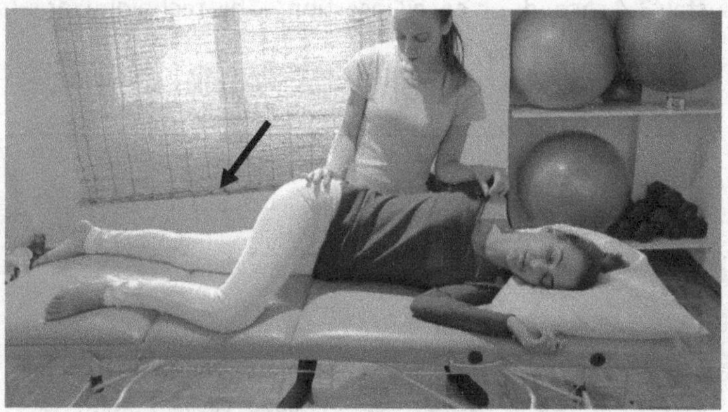

62. Put the receiver's arm behind your back, and place your hand next to the hip joint. Push the hip joint forwards, taking care not to put pressure on the shoulder.

This technique targets the lower lumbar vertebrae, and is indicated for sciatica and lower back pain.

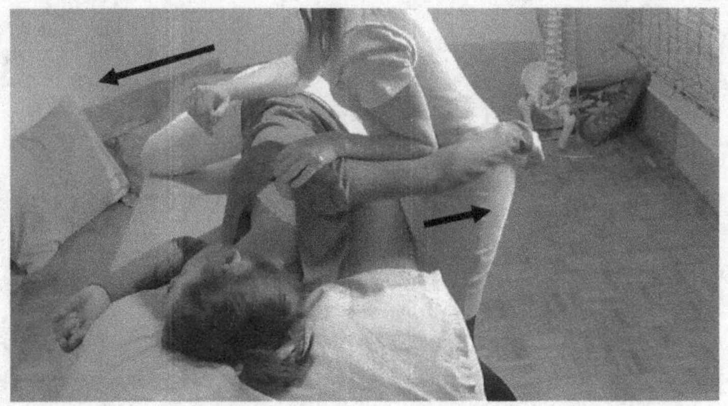

63. Same technique as before, but executed with the forearm for better leverage.

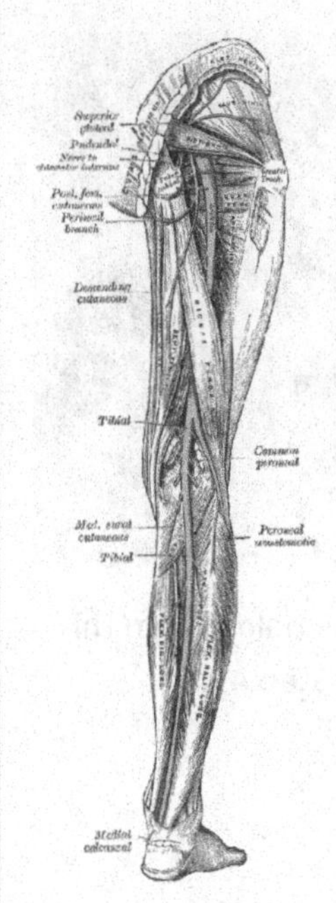

The sciatic nerve

The sciatic nerve begins in the lower back and runs through the buttock and down the lower limb. It is the longest and widest single nerve in the human body, going from the top of the leg to the foot on the posterior aspect.

The sciatic nerve provides the connection to the nervous system for nearly the whole of the skin of the leg, the muscles of the back of the thigh, and those of the leg and foot. It is derived from spinal nerves L4 to S3.

Pain caused by a compression or irritation of the sciatic nerve by a problem in the lower back is called sciatica. Common causes of sciatica include the following lower back and hip conditions: spinal disc herniation, degenerative disc disease, lumbar spinal stenosis, spondylolisthesis, and piriformis syndrome.

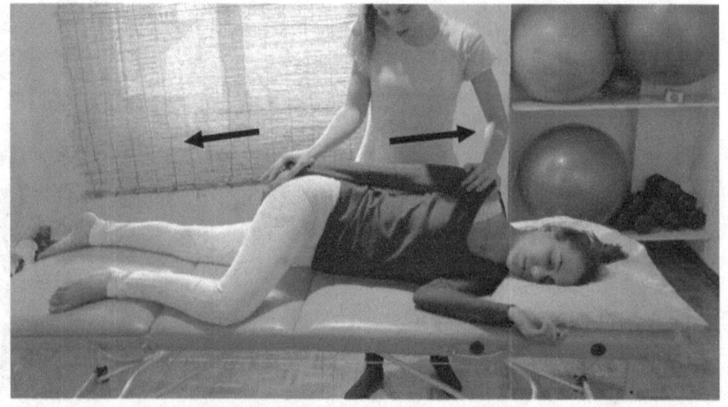

64. Then stretch the arm, and do Jap Sen work on the outer arm, on the Itha & Pingkala branch. It is recommended to work on the dorsal surface of the hand as well, on the Sen lines.

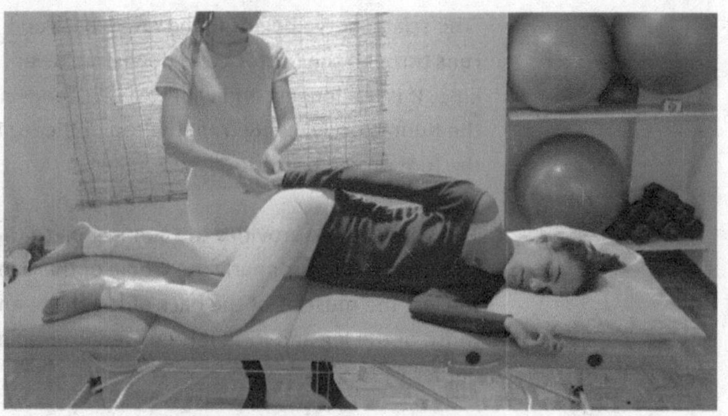

65. Rotate the hand in order to expose the palm. From this position, you can apply the techniques of Step 47.

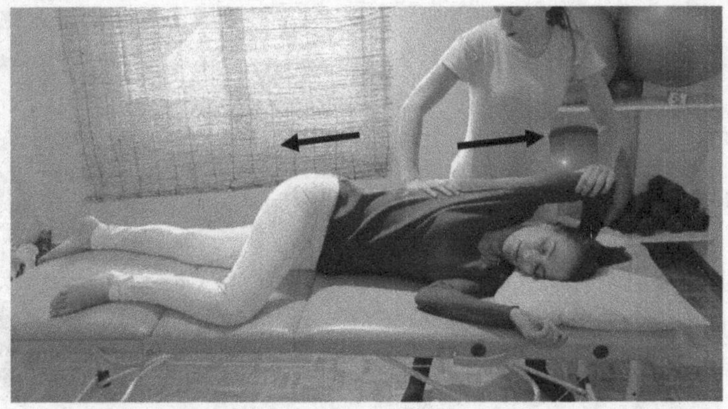

66. Place the arm in the "triangle" position (fingers facing the shoulder, bent arm) and stretch the torso. Start "opening" the ribs, thus creating space in the thoracic cage.

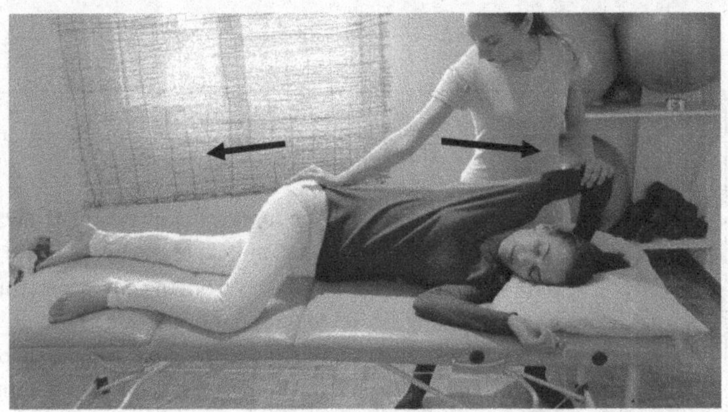

67. With the bent arm still locked, place your palm above the receiver's pelvis and stretch the lateral side of the torso.

This and the previous technique are more effective at the side position (rather than in the supine), because now the therapist can access a much larger part of the torso. They are recommended for upper back pain, kyphosis, scoliosis and breathing problems.

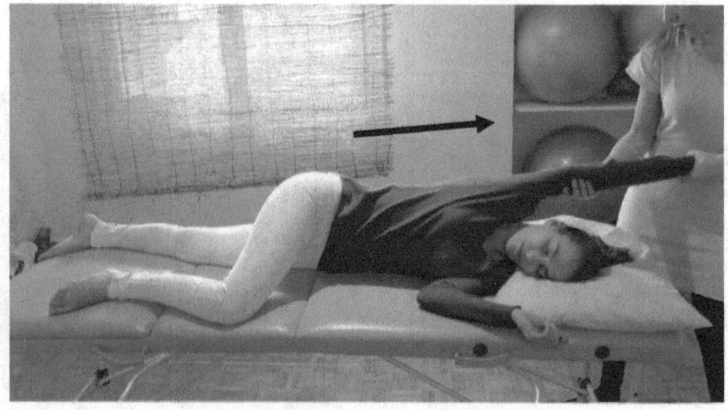

68. Grasp the receiver's arm, and pull it backwards, in order to open the ribs and the thoracic spine.

Do not apply this technique, or steps 67 and 66 if the client has unstable shoulder joint and / or supraspinatus injury.

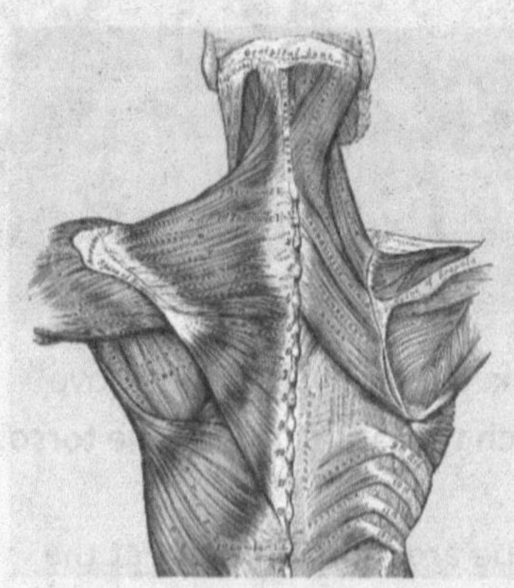

The supraspinatus

The supraspinatus is a relatively small muscle of the upper back that runs from the supraspinatous fossa superior portion of the scapula to the greater tubercle of the humerus. It is one of the four rotator cuff muscles and also abducts the arm at the shoulder.

Tears are common, and usually due to repetitive stress. If the client has a supraspinatus injury, avoid mobilizations that place the arm above the head, and also intense lateral pulling of the arm.

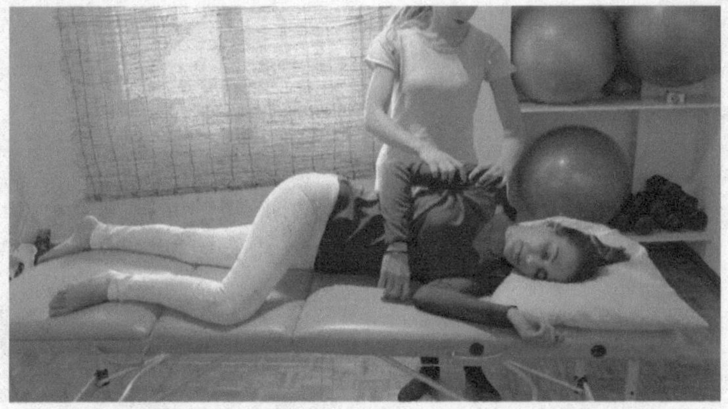

69. Massage the deltoid muscle – a must for any type of shoulder pain.

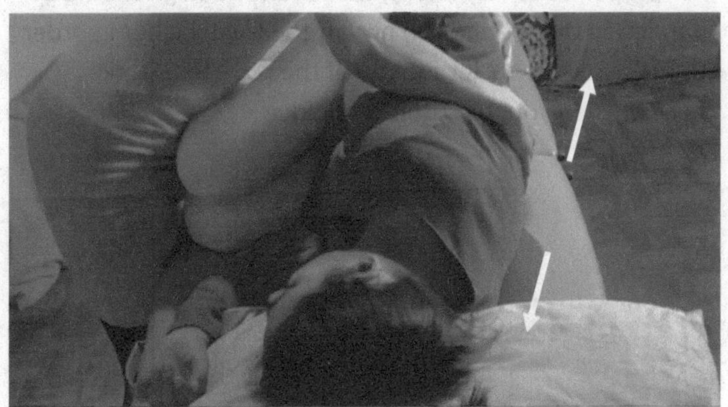

70. Bend the client's legs and place them on your belly. Start mobilizing them forth and back, in order to relax the lower back. Then, create a stretch on the lower back with your hands: place one hand on the sacrum, and one hand at the beginning of the lumbar spine, while pushing the receiver's legs upwards, towards her head.

This technique is possible only on the table – you cannot do it on the floor.

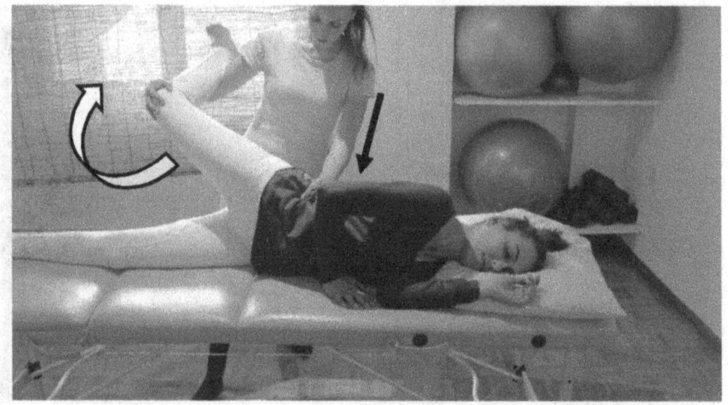

71. Grasp the patella and stretch the leg backwards. Place your hand on the lower back for stability.

For proper body alignment, the receiver's thigh should be parallel to the ground. Do not lift the thigh higher in order to make the lift easier for you. If the receiver is much heavier than you, omit this technique.

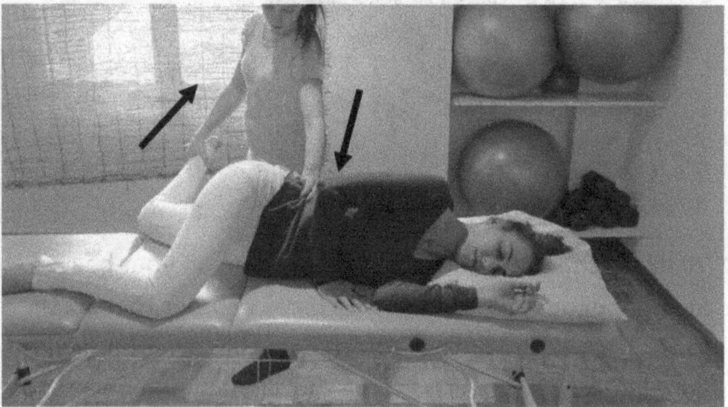

72. Same as before, but in this technique I am stretching the other leg.

Do not overdo the stretching in this and in the previous technique, and be cautious if the client has a slipped disc.

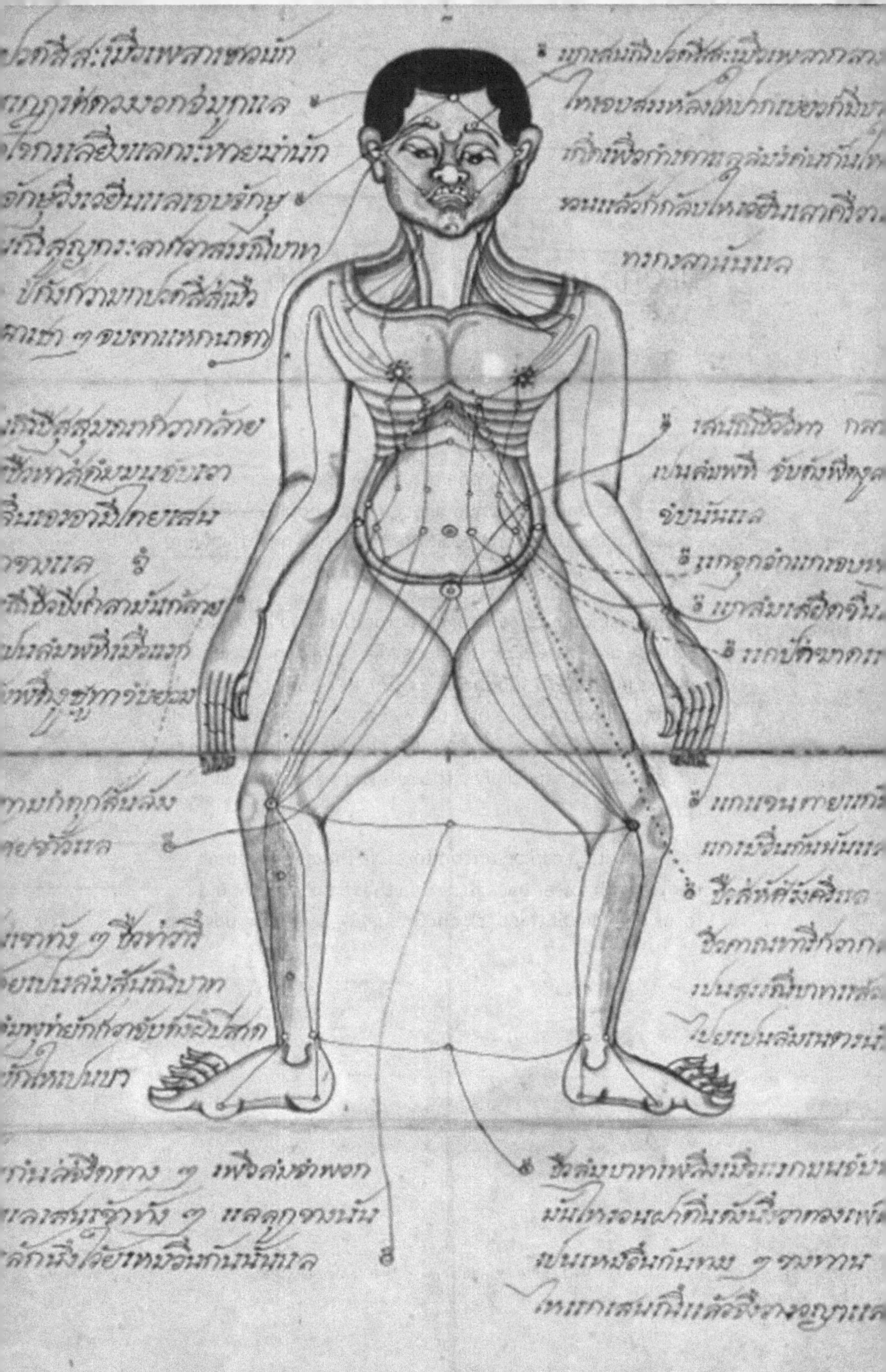

Prone position

efinitely, the prone position is the most relaxing massage position. In fact, most people have in mind the prone position when they hear the word "massage" – it is something like a synonym.

Prone position is of course, great for back and legs massage, as these areas are directly exposed. You may need some pillows in order to support the receiver's body properly. You may have to place one pillow under the receiver's belly, in case of lumbar lordosis. A pillow under the lower legs can also be useful, especially if the receiver has externally rotated legs.

Prone position can be uncomfortable though, for some people with lower back issues. In that case, you should focus on work at the back and the legs, in the side position.

Techniques in prone position

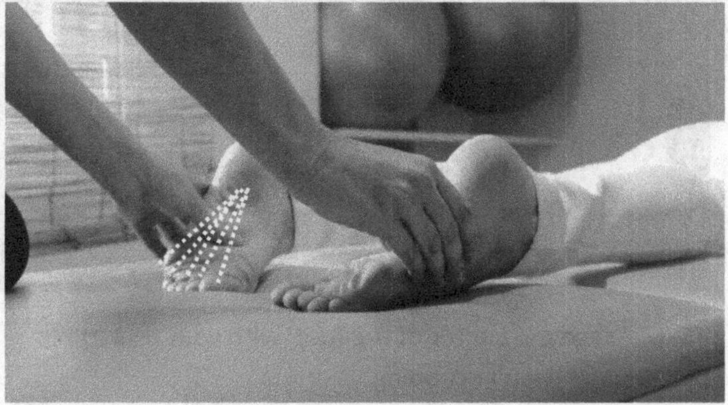

73. Start at the feet. Press the Kalatharee Sen lines on the feet. Work from the heel towards the toes, and from the big toe towards the 5th toe.

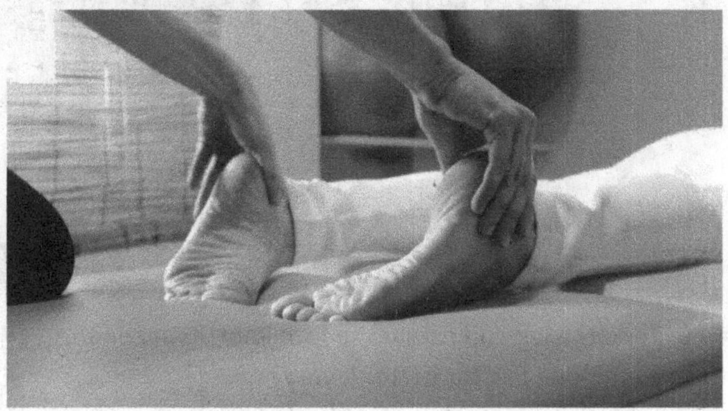

74. Massage and rub the heels. Work at both feet simultaneously.

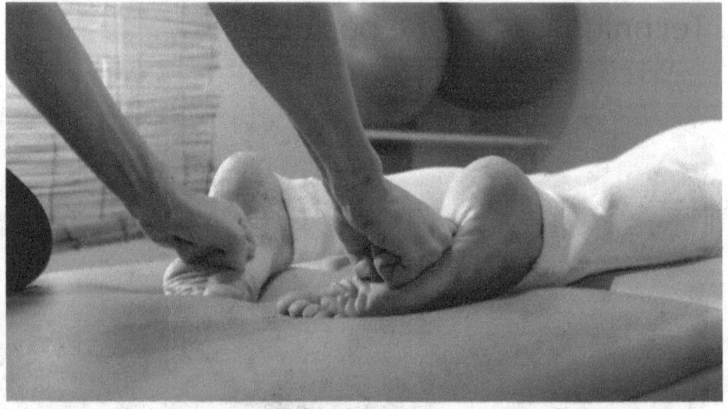

75. Massage the center of the foot, with your fists. Do presses and circular rubbing.

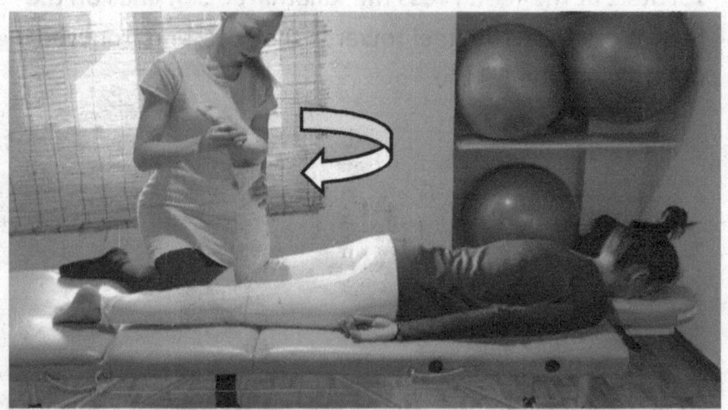

76. Bend the leg and rotate the foot joint. Kneel on the table with one leg, for better leverage.
Do 5 rotations on each foot, at both directions.

From this technique, and up to step 85, kneel with one leg on the table, for better leverage.

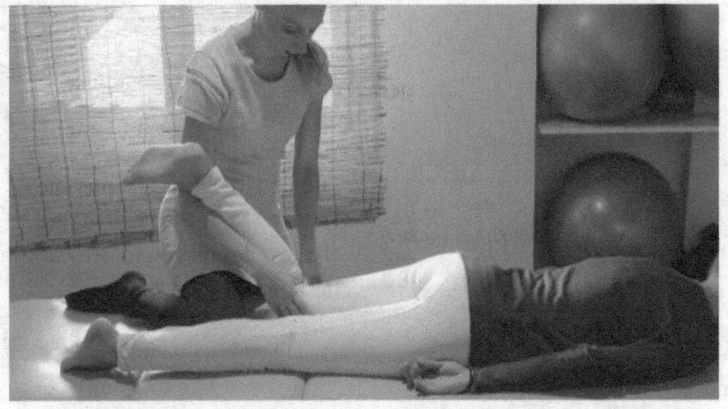

77. Work in the popliteal fossa with your thumbs, VERY gently. Lift the receiver's leg and place it on your arms in order to do this. NEVER work in this area without bending the leg!
This is an Itha & Pingkala acupressure point, for knee and lower back pain. It is on the same spot with Chinese acupoint UB40, which has similar indications.

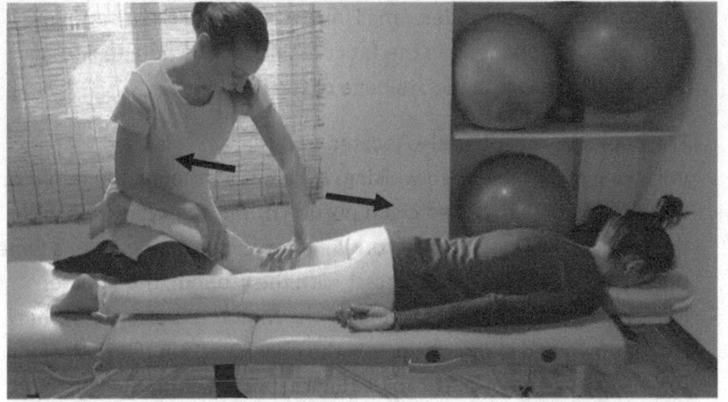

78. Place the receiver's lower leg on your thigh, and stretch the popliteal area. This is indicated for knee pain. The stretch also affects the popliteus, gastrocnemius and biceps femoris muscles.

The popliteal fossa

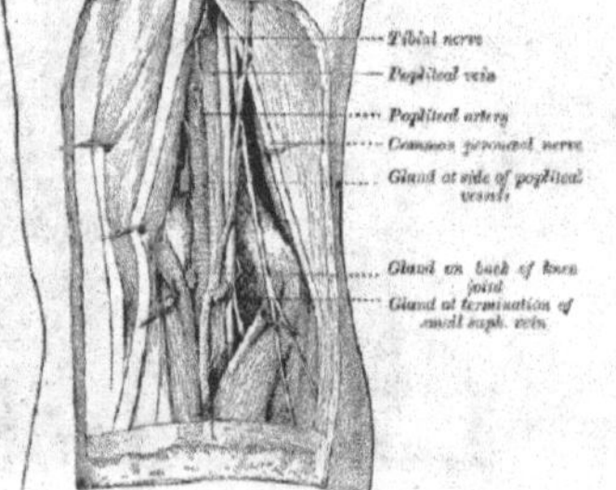

The popliteal fossa (sometimes referred to as the kneepit) is a shallow depression located at the back of the knee joint.

Structures within the popliteal fossa include, (from superficial to deep):

- tibial nerve
- common peroneal nerve
- popliteal vein
- popliteal artery, a continuation of the femoral artery
- small saphenous vein (termination)
- Popliteal lymph nodes

The popliteal lymph nodes, small in size and some six or seven in number, are embedded in the fat contained in the popliteal fossa. They assist the lymphatic drainage of the legs.

The popliteus muscle is also located in this area. It is used for unlocking the knees when walking, by laterally rotating the femur on the tibia during the closed chain portion of the gait cycle (one with the foot in contact with the ground). In open chain movements (when the involved limb is not in contact with the ground), the popliteus muscle medially rotates the tibia on the femur. It is also used when sitting down and standing up. It is the only muscle in the posterior (back) compartment of the lower leg that acts just on the knee and not on the ankle.

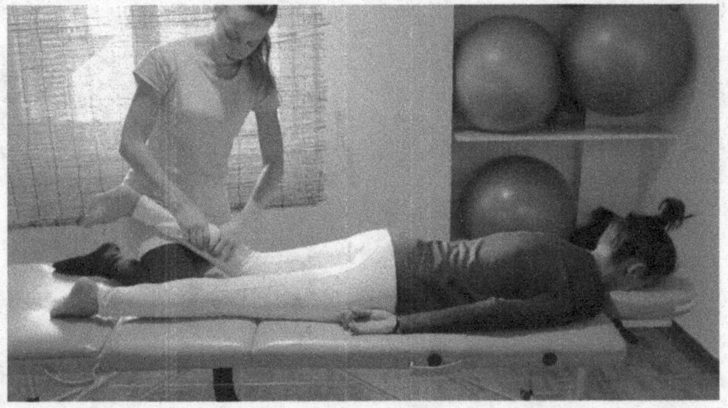

79. With the receiver's lower leg still on your thigh, massage the calf muscle.

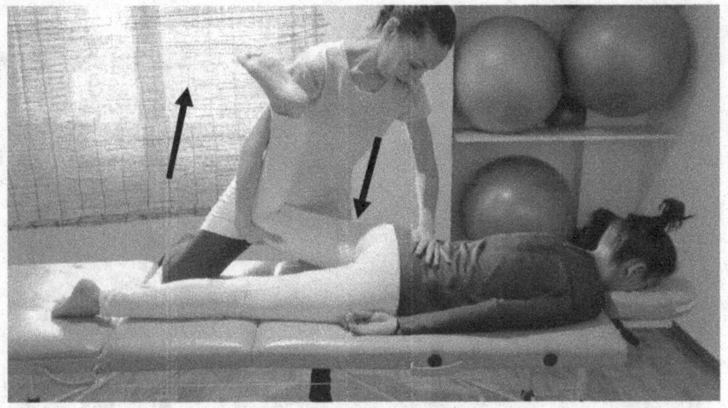

80. Lift the leg by holding it from the patella, and stabilize the lower back with your palm. Omit this step if the client has lordosis, degenerative disc disease or spinal stenosis.

This technique has similarities with the typical orthopedic Femoral Nerve Stretch test or Mackiewicz sign – if it is positive (that is, if the receiver experiences pain at the lumbar spine) it may mean that the nerves in the 3rd – 4th lumbar vertebrae are compressed.

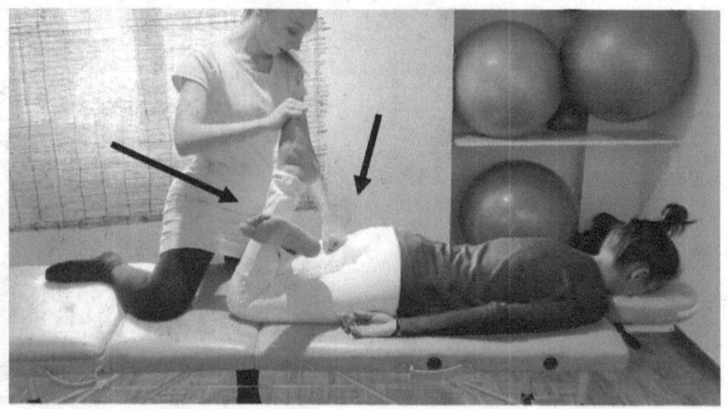

81. Press the posterior thigh muscles with your fist, while pushing the lower leg. This technique is indicated for sciatica.

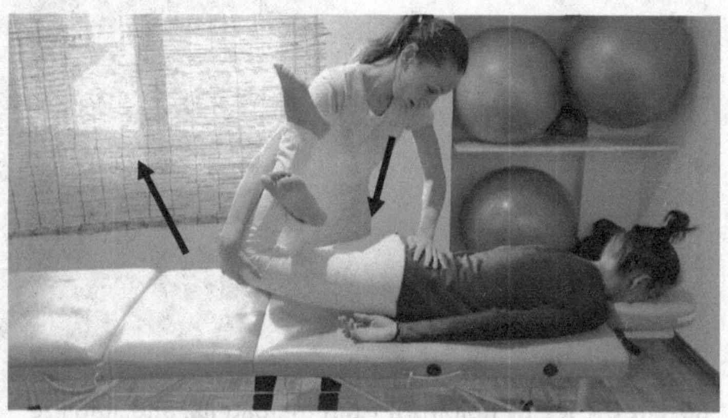

82. Lift the leg by holding it from the patella, and stabilize the lower back with your palm. This stretches the quadriceps muscle.

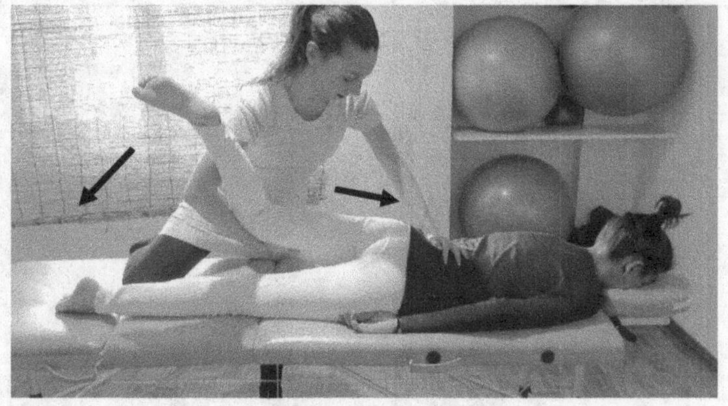

83. Grasp the leg and rotate it slightly inwards, while pushing on the lumbar spine upwards. This decompresses the lower back.

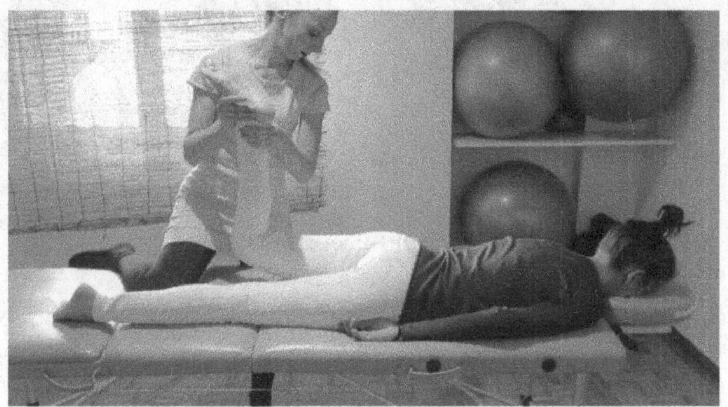

84. Lift the leg, and shake it gently.

Repeat on the other leg all the techniques from step 76 until this step.

Muscles of the posterior leg

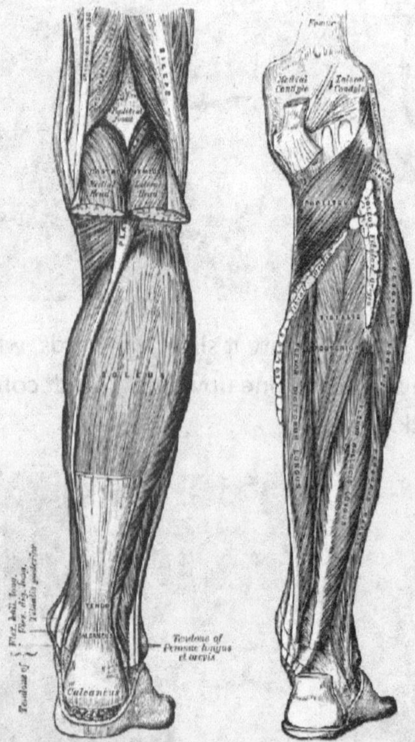

Of the posterior muscles three are in the superficial layer.

The major plantar flexors are:

- the soleus, which arises on the proximal side of both leg bones
- the gastrocnemius, the two heads of which arises on the distal end of the femur.

These muscles unite in a large terminal tendon, the Achilles tendon, which is attached to the posterior tubercle of the calcaneus.

The plantaris closely follows the lateral head of the gastrocnemius. Its tendon runs between those of the soleus and gastrocnemius and is embedded in the medial end of the calcaneus tendon.

In the deep layer:

- The tibialis posterior has its origin on the interosseus membrane and the neighboring bone areas and runs down behind the medial malleolus. Under the foot it splits into a thick medial part attached to the navicular bone and a slightly weaker lateral part inserted to the three cuneiform bones. The muscle produces simultaneous plantar flexion and supination in the non-weight-bearing leg, and approximates the heel to the calf of the leg.

- The flexor hallucis longus arises distally on the fibula and on the interosseus membrane from where its relatively thick muscle belly extends far distally. Its tendon extends beneath the flexor retinaculum to the sole of the foot and finally attaches on the base of the last phalanx of the hallux. It plantarflexes the hallux and assists in supination.

- The flexor digitorum longus, finally, has its origin on the upper part of the tibia. Its tendon runs to the sole of the foot where it forks into four terminal tendon attached to the last phalanges of the four lateral toes. It crosses the tendon of the tibialis posterior distally on the tibia, and the tendon of the flexor hallucis longus in the sole.

- Distally to its division, the quadratus plantae radiates into it and near the middle phalanges its tendons penetrate the tendons of the flexor digitorum brevis. In the non-weight-bearing leg, it plantar flexes the toes and foot and supinates. In the weight-bearing leg it supports the plantar arch.

The presses and the stretches of Thai Massage can help to ease leg pain and improve athletic function. They can also be used in rehabilitation after injuries.

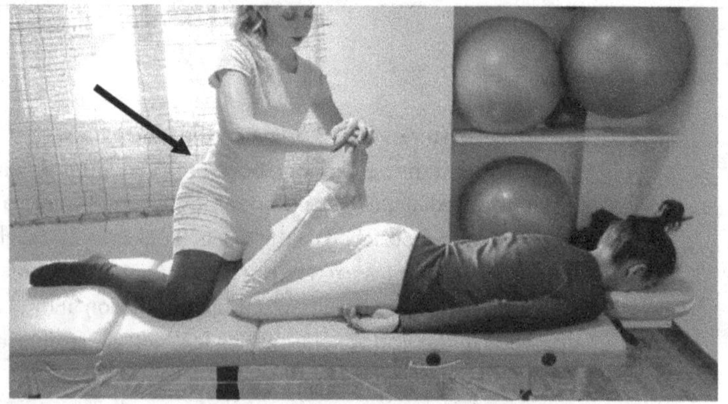

85. Cross the feet and push them towards the client's sacrum. Do not overdo it, and avoid it in people with lordosis, degenerative disc disease or spinal stenosis.

Omit steps 80-85 if there is any knee injury.

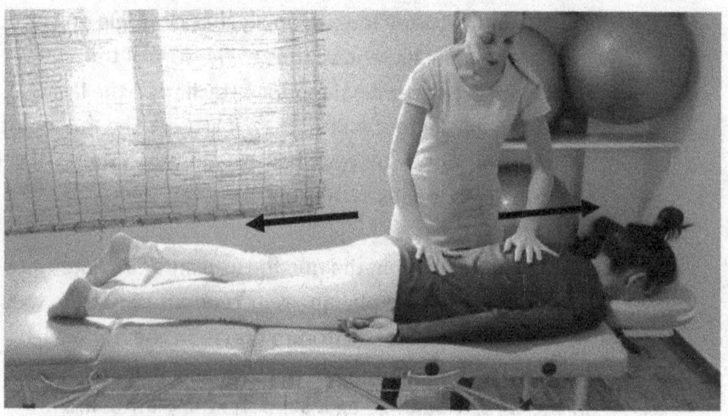

86. Yes! We'll start working on the back!

Begin with a light stretch. Place one hand on the lumbar spine, and one hand on the thoracic spine, and stretch. The center of your palm should be on the spinous processes.

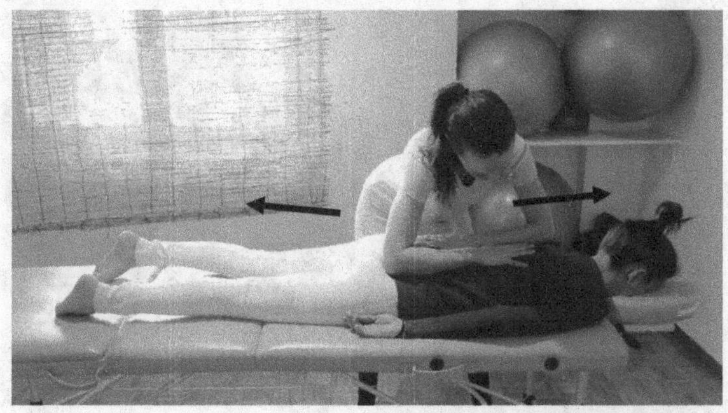

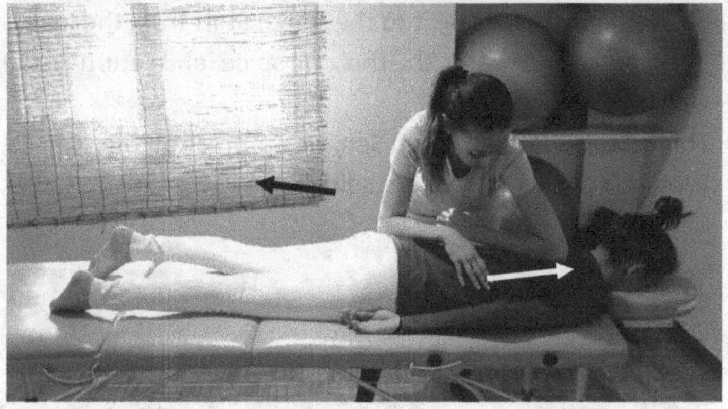

87. I'll do Jap Sen on the back, on the Itha & Pingkala posterior branches.

Begin with four stretches on the back, using your forearms. Important: Do not press with your elbow joint, it will be painful!

Place one forearm next to the shoulder blade, and one on the gluteus muscle. Upon exhalation, use your body weight in order to apply the stretch.

Do four stretches on the back – two one the same side, and two on opposite sides.

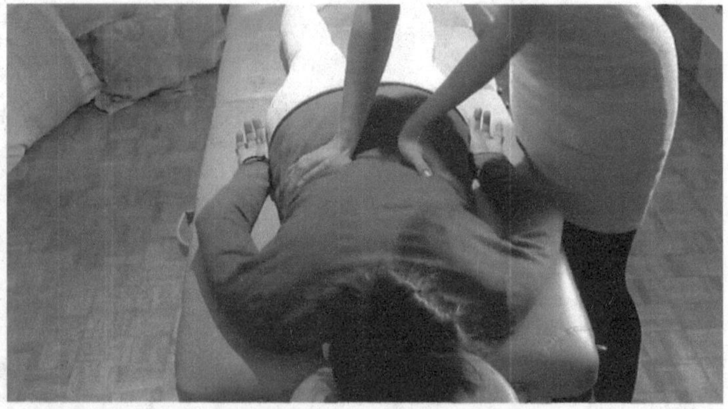

88. Do palm presses next to the spine. Start from the lower back, proceed towards the thoracic spine, and return all the way down.
This is Step 2 (and 4) of Jap Sen. Never press on the scapula. Work 1.5 cm away from the spine.

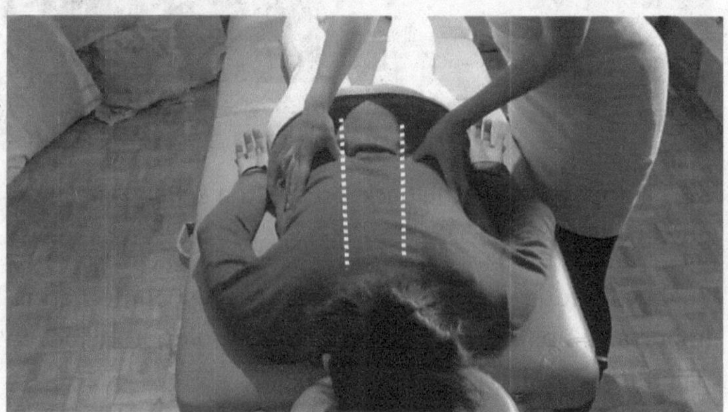

89. Then do thumb presses on the Itha & Pingkala Sen lines on the back. Work your way up the 7th cervical vertebra. Work on acupressure points on the lower back or between the shoulder blades, as needed.
Then repeat the palm presses (step 88) and the stretches (step 87) in order to complete the Jap Sen protocol.

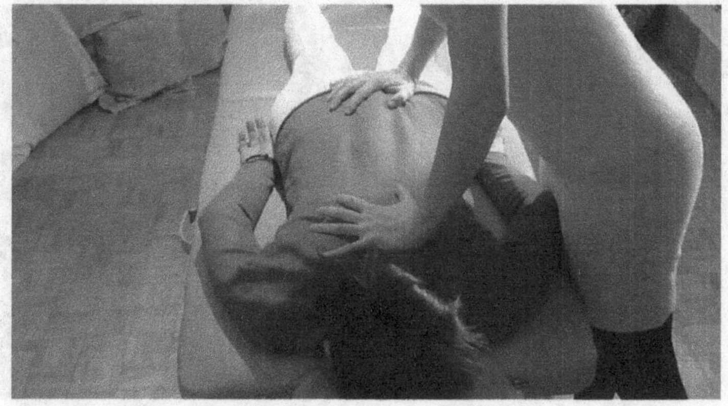

90. Do another light stretch on the back...

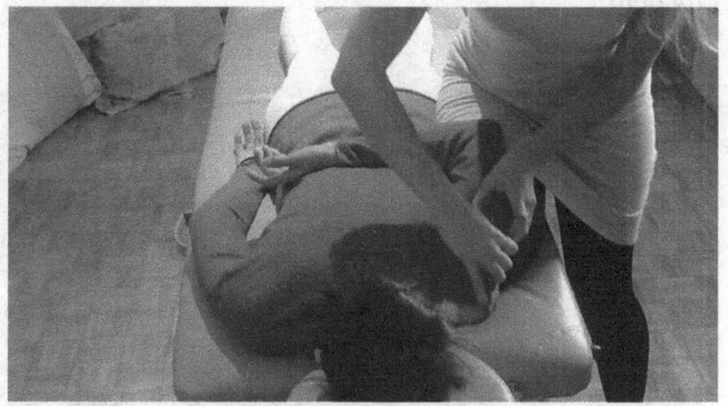

91. And start massaging the deltoid and the biceps muscle.
In order to do this efficiently, bend the receiver's arm and
place the forearm on the back.
I prefer to place my thigh on the table, and support the
receiver's arm on it, for better leverage.

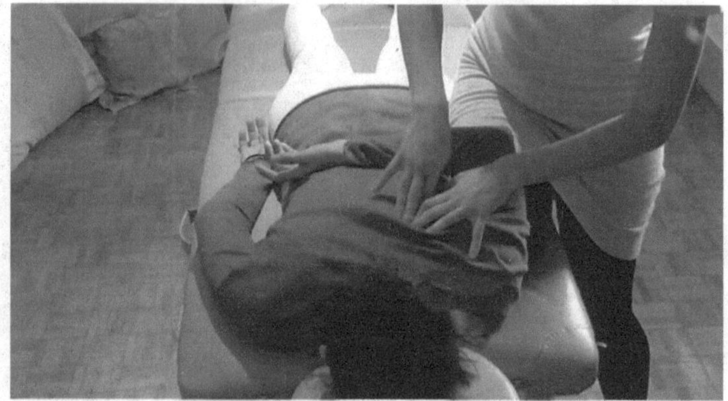

92. Still in the same position, work next to the shoulder blade. Do circular friction and deep tissue (transverse friction).

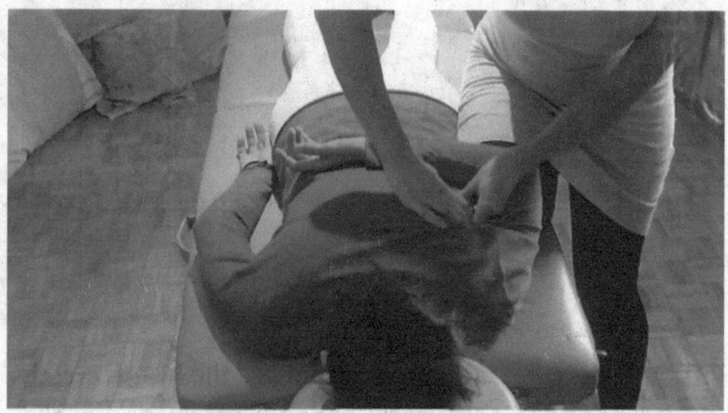

93. Do skin rolling (yes, it can be done as a dry massage technique, and above clothing!) on the teres major muscle.

This is a small muscle, and it assists the action of the very large latissimus dorsi muscle.

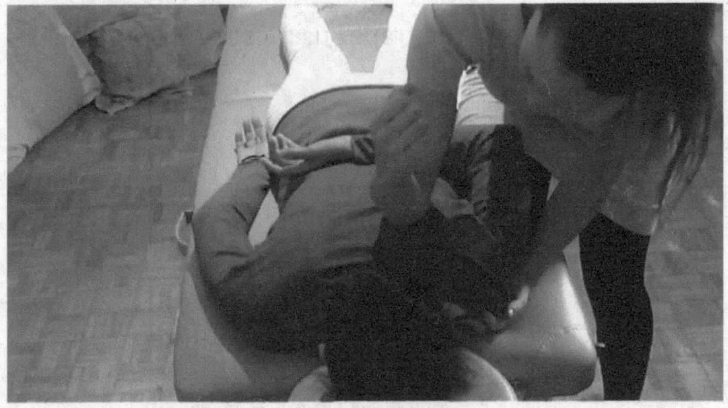

94. You can use your elbow, but be careful not to press too strongly, unless the client is much larger than you, or asks for strong work.
Actually, the elbow can be a quite precise tool, and is always valuable in dry massage. Use it only after warming properly the tissues.

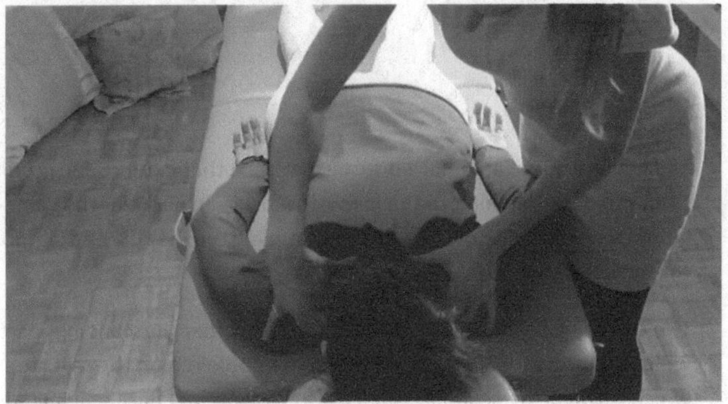

95. Do kneading massage on the trapezius muscle. This is the typical Swedish massage kneading, and works great as a dry massage technique as well. If you find any tender spots (we all have those there!) do more work on this area.

The trapezius muscle

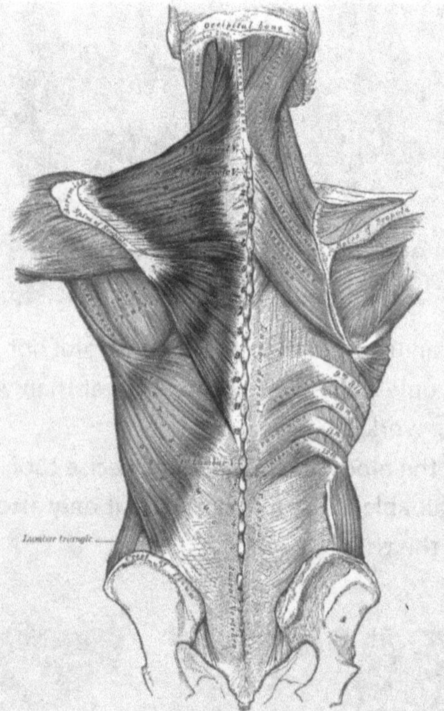

The trapezius is a large paired surface muscle that extends longitudinally from the occipital bone to the lower thoracic vertebrae of the spine and laterally to the spine of the scapula. It moves the scapula and supports the arm.

The trapezius has three functional parts: an upper (descending) part which supports the weight of the arm; a middle region (transverse), which retracts the scapula; and a lower (ascending) part which medially rotates and depresses the scapula.

Muscular tensions that produce upper back pain, are very common in the trapezius muscle, and are usually due to bad postural habits. Massage helps a lot. I recommend adding hot herbal packs on this muscle, before and after the application of massage therapy.

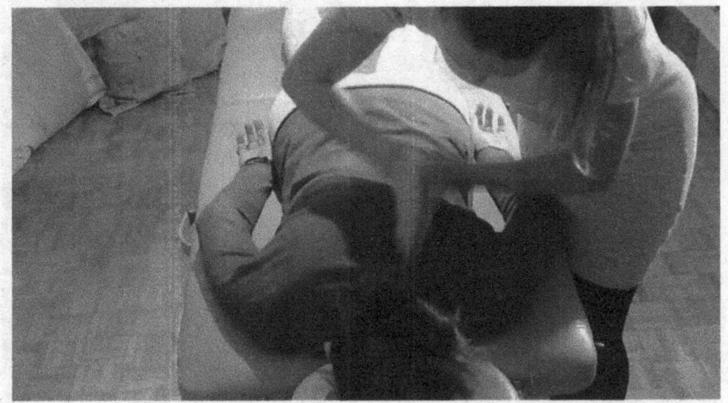

96. Continue with the tapping technique known as the "Thai Slap". This technique, like all tapping (known also as tapotement) techniques improve the circulation of the blood and the lymph. Repeat 5 times on each shoulder.

How to do the Thai Slap Technique

This is one of the most characteristic tapotement techniques of Thai Massage.

In order to perform it properly:

1. Join palms.

2. Keep fingers apart.

3. Maintain loose wrists - Release all tension from your wrists.

4. Join the heels of your hands - however, do not join the wrist joints.

5. Then, let your hands fall, performing the slap. You should hear the typical clapping sound.

It is important to let go of all tension throughout the technique. Never perform this kind of work over bony areas.

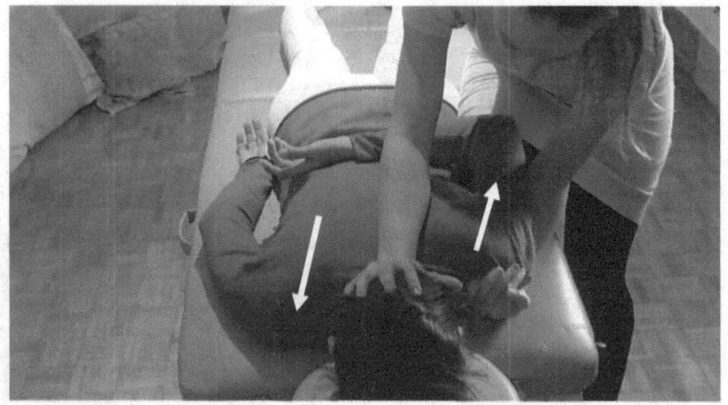

97. Hold the shoulder and pull it, while pushing gently the head upwards from the occipital bone. Wonderful technique for upper back pain.

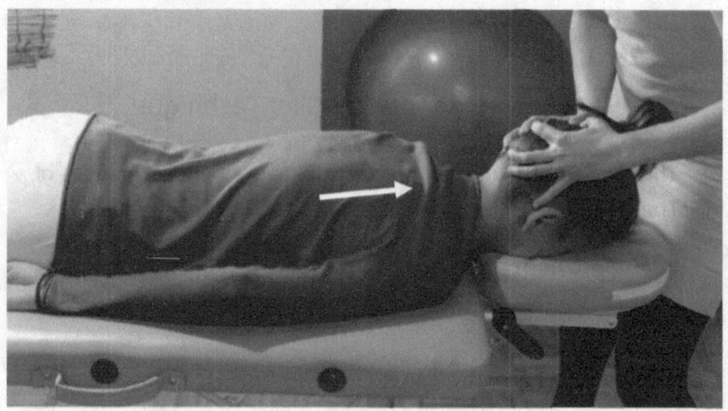

98. Pull the head in order to decompress the neck. This pulling should be done at a horizontal axis – never push the receiver's head on the armrest.

it is recommended to do rubbing work on the atlanto-occipital joint from this position, as this area has valuable acupressure points for headaches.

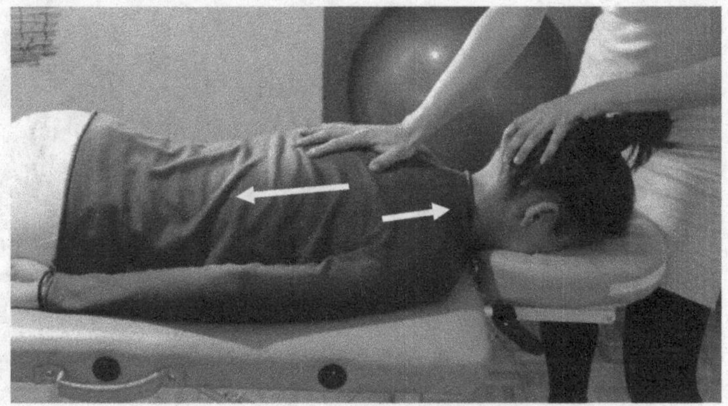

99. Pull the occipital bone, while pushing gently the spine towards the feet. In this occasion too, you should work at a horizontal axis, at both hands.

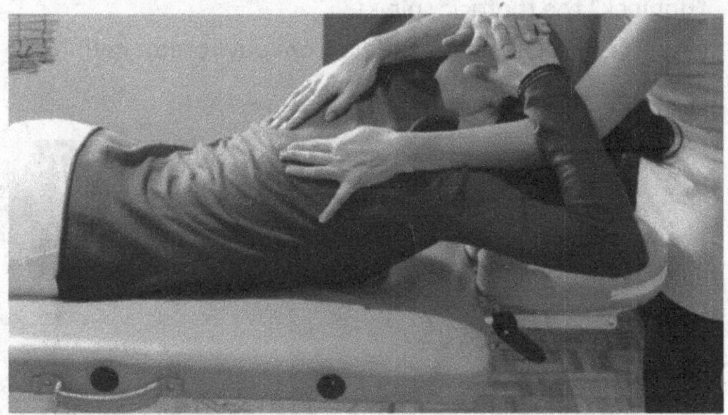

100. Ask the client to interlock her fingers behind her head, and place your hands on the thoracic spine. Lift the torso. From this lock, you can also rotate and stretch gently the torso.
This technique is indicated for tension and imbalances at the thoracic spine. Its effect is like the one of the "Cobra" posture in traditional Thai Massage on the floor. However, this technique does not stress the lumbar spine.

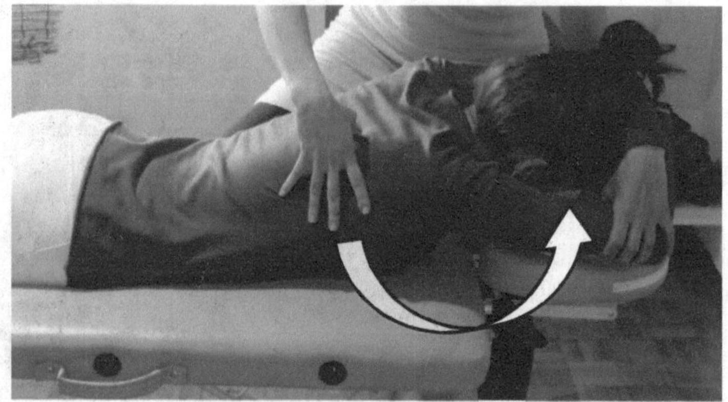

101. Ask the client to lay one arm on the other as shown. Grasp her arms with one hand (place it under the interlocked arms), and with your other hand work on the thoracic spine. You can also rotate the torso, in order to "unblock" the thoracic spine.
Omit this if the receiver suffers from any rotator cuff injury.

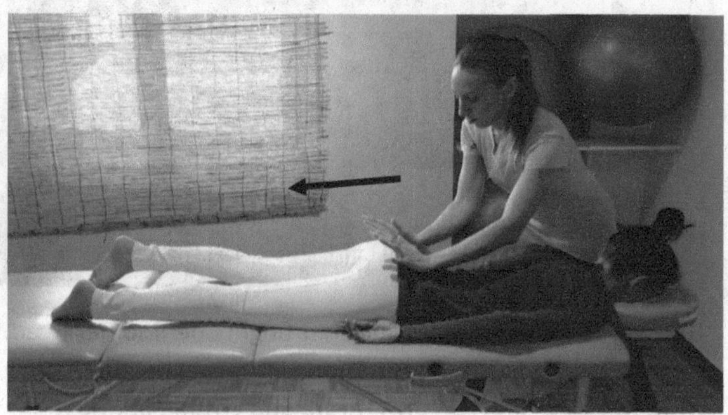

102. Place your hands on the top of the gluteus muscles, and push the muscles downwards, towards the receiver's feet. This decompresses the lumbar spine.

This concludes the prone position.

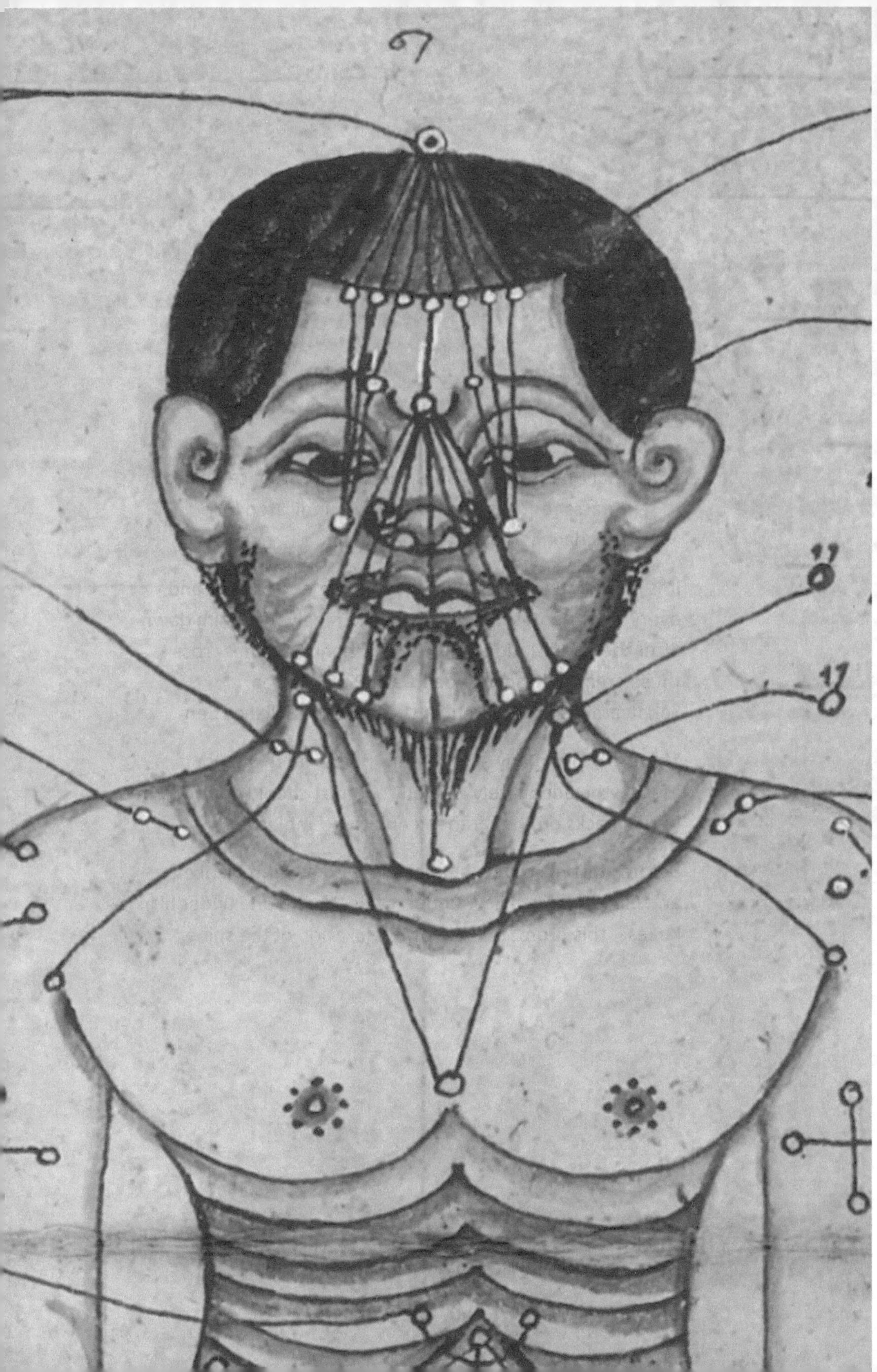

Face and scalp

Thai Massage session is concluded with face and scalp massage. These techniques are indicated for headaches, stress and neck pain.

It is recommended to apply them in the end of each and every treatment, since they help the receiver to calm down after the mobilizations. Moreover, many Sen lines cross these areas – these include Itha & Pingkala Sen, Sahatsarangsi & Tawaree Sen, Lawusang & Ulanga Sen.

There are also many acupressure points on the head. Ideally, the adequately trained therapist should apply warm herbal packs on the forehead and the temples.

Before starting, cover the receiver with a warm blanket, and place a large pillow under his head, and one under his knees – this promotes the total relaxation of the spine.

Relaxing the shoulders and the scalp

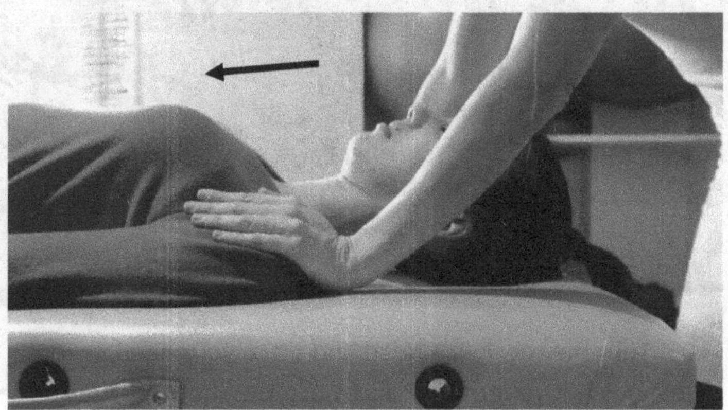

103. Start by pushing down the shoulders alternatively. Work gently and slowly. Repeat 4-5 times.

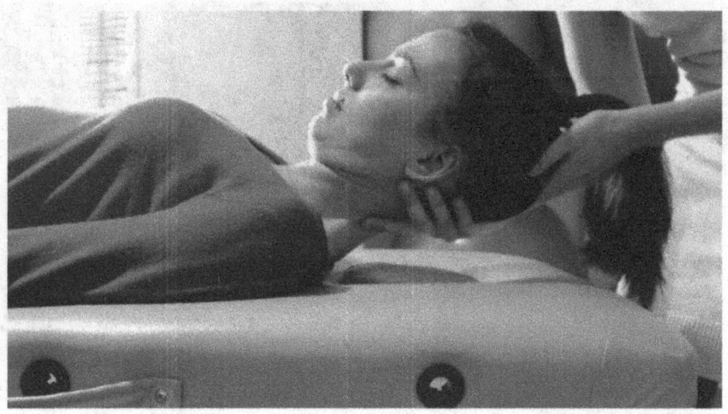

104. Slide your hands on the neck alternatively. Your hands should reach until the occipital bone. Pull gently the head each time you pass from the occipital bone.

It is recommended to slide your hands as far as possible down to the trapezius muscle, for maximum relaxation.

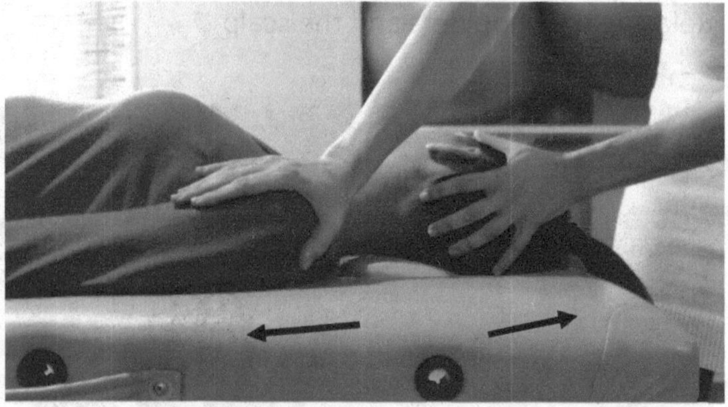

105. Turn the receiver's head and place your hand next to the ear. With your other hand, push the shoulder towards the feet.

Repeat on the other side. Take care NOT to push the head in this technique - push only the shoulder.

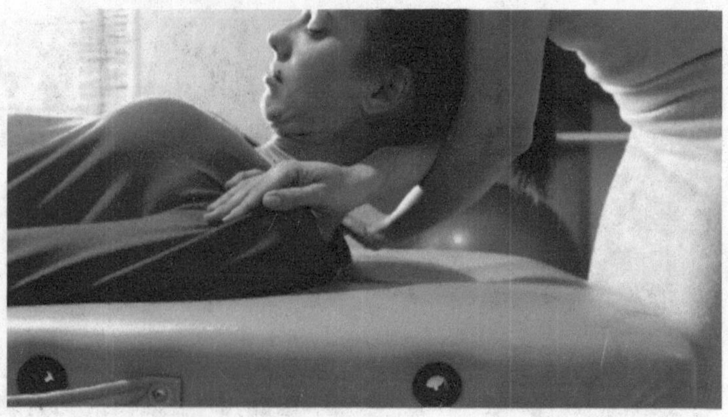

106. Cross your arms behind the client's neck, and lift her head while pressing gently the shoulders. Hold the stretch for 5-10 seconds.

Omit this technique in clients with degenerated discs at the cervical spine.

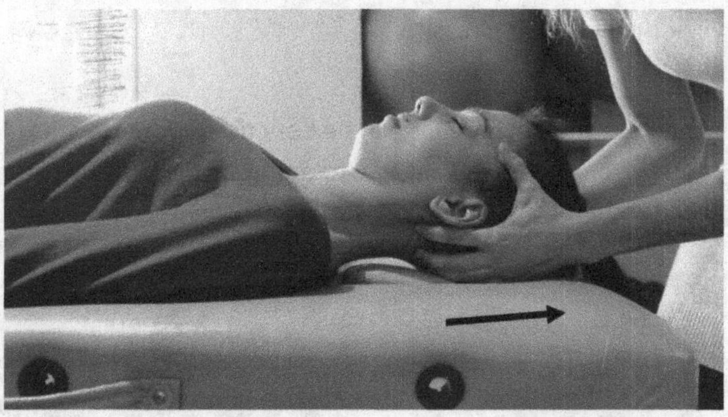

107. Grasp the atlanto-occipital joint, and pull the head. This technique can release the recti capitis posteriores major and minor, and the obliquus capitis superior muscles, which are often involved in headaches.

Atlanto-occipital joint and headaches

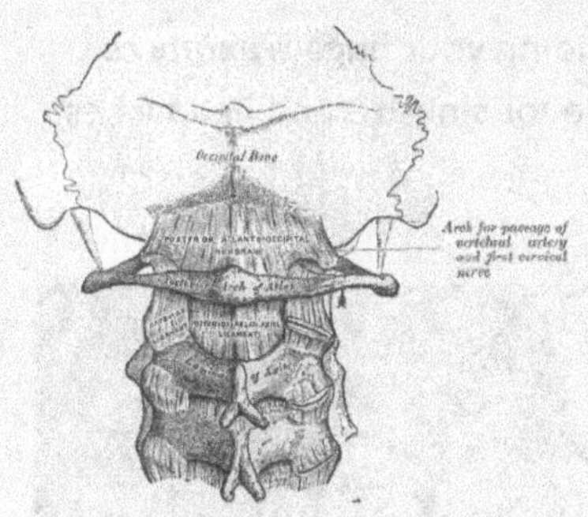

The atlanto-occipital joint is the articulation between the atlas and the occipital bone. The movements permitted in this joint are:
(a) flexion and extension around the mediolateral axis, which give rise to the ordinary forward and backward nodding of the head.
(b) slight lateral motion, lateroflexion, to one or other side around the anteroposterior axis.

Flexion is produced mainly by the action of the longi capitis and recti capitis anteriores; extension by the recti capitis posteriores major and minor, the obliquus capitis superior, the semispinalis capitis, splenius capitis, sternocleidomastoideus, and upper fibers of the trapezius.

There is a definite correlation between chronic headaches and the rectus capitis muscles, especially in suboccipital headaches.

Techniques for sinusitis

The following techniques can be beneficial for those who
suffer from sinusitis. Feel free to apply strong pressure on
the forehead.

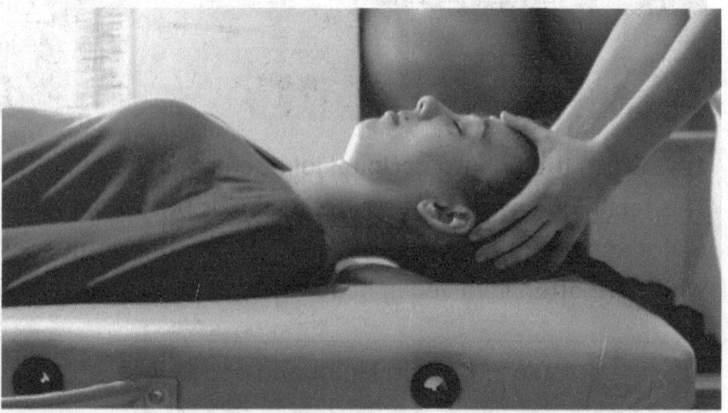

108. Work on the forehead, sliding your fingers gently but
firmly. This is a good technique for sinusitis and headaches.

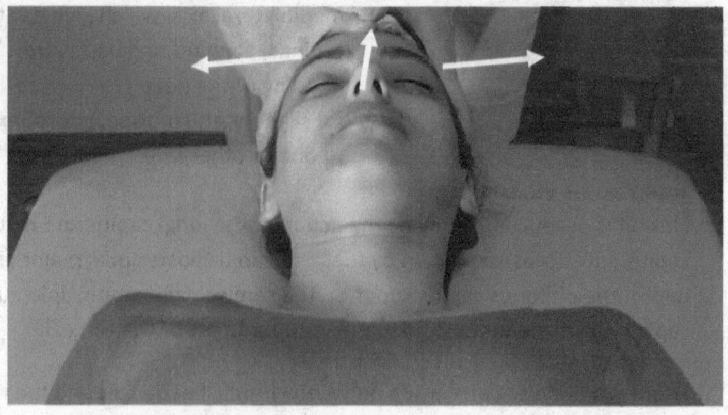

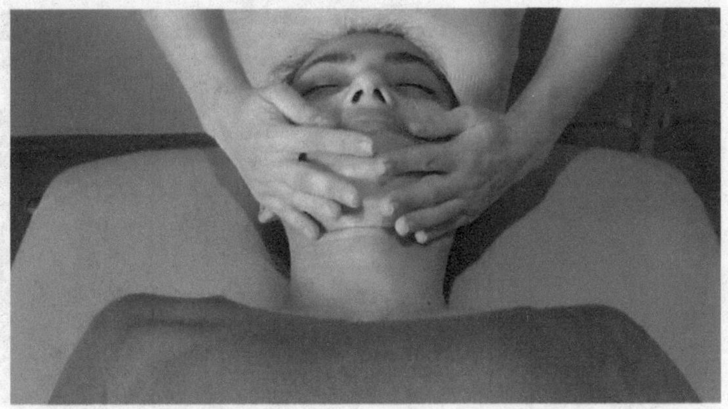

109. Place your thumbs above the lips, and your index fingers below the lips, and pull the face...

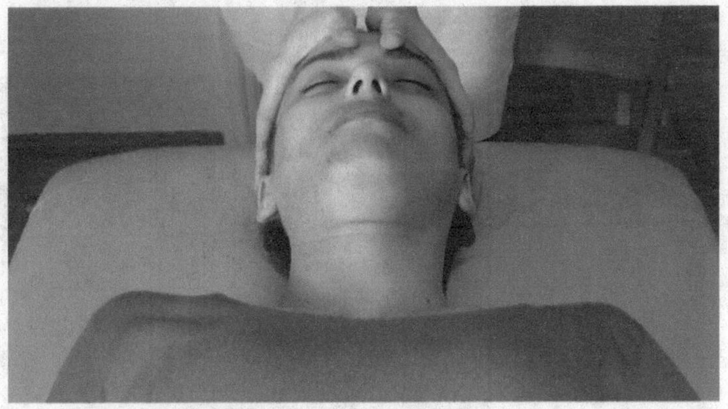

110... then slide your thumbs on the forehead.

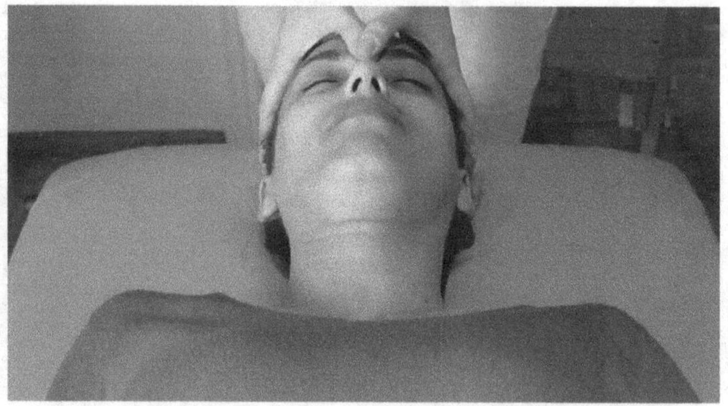

111. Press three points, from the root of the nose up to the hairline.

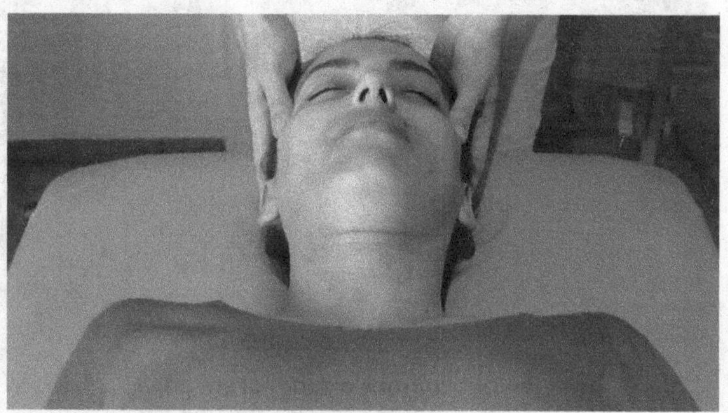

112. Press three points right below the hairline, and then rub the temples.

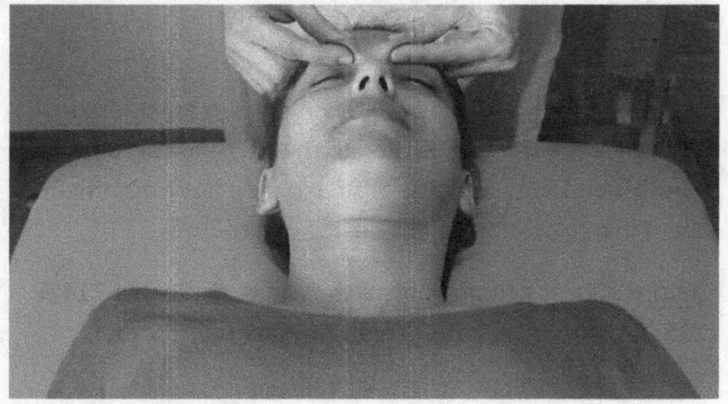

113. Pinch the eyebrows. The first point targets the Corrugator supercilii muscle.

The corrugator supercilii muscle

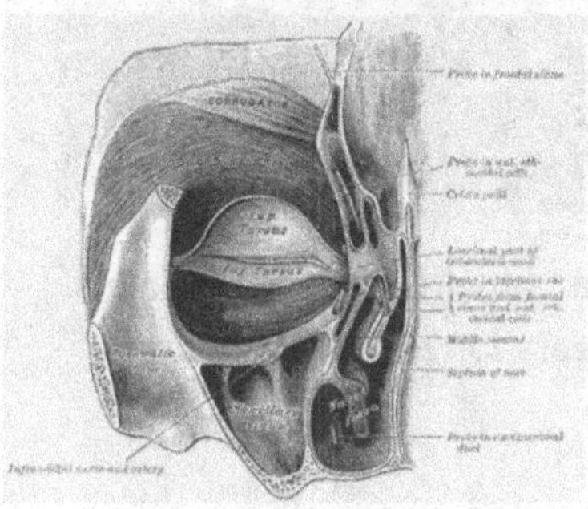

The corrugator supercilii is a small, narrow, pyramidal muscle close to the eye. It is located at the medial end of the eyebrow.

The corrugator draws the eyebrow downward and medially, producing the vertical wrinkles of the forehead.

It is the "frowning" muscle, and may be regarded as the principal muscle in the expression of suffering. It also contracts to prevent high sun glare, pulling the eyebrows toward the bridge of the nose, making a roof over the area above the middle corner of the eye and typical forehead furrows.

This muscle can store a lot of tension because of stress.

Ear massage techniques

I learned the three following techniques in my traditional Thai Massage training. Although they are indicated for sinusitis and for lymphatic drainage, I do not recommend them in a relaxation treatment.

Before applying them, inform the client. Omit step 114 & 115 in clients that suffer from any inner ear disorder.

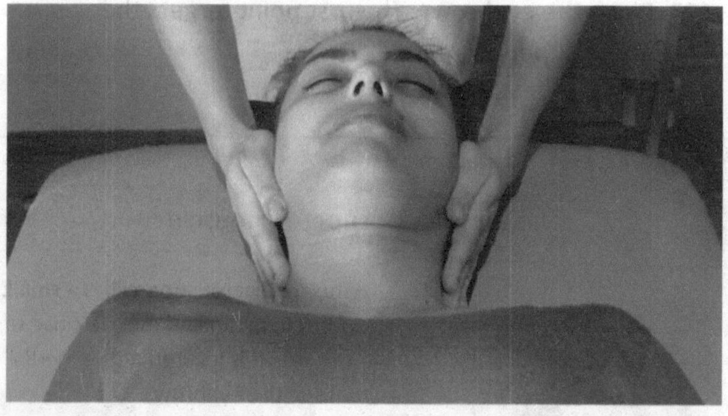

114. Cover the ears, and make a half-circle with your palms. Push gently your palms on the ears for 10-15 seconds, and release.

If you do this correctly, you will hear a strong clapping sound upon the release. Clients who have closed their eyes during the massage session, open them suddenly upon the release.

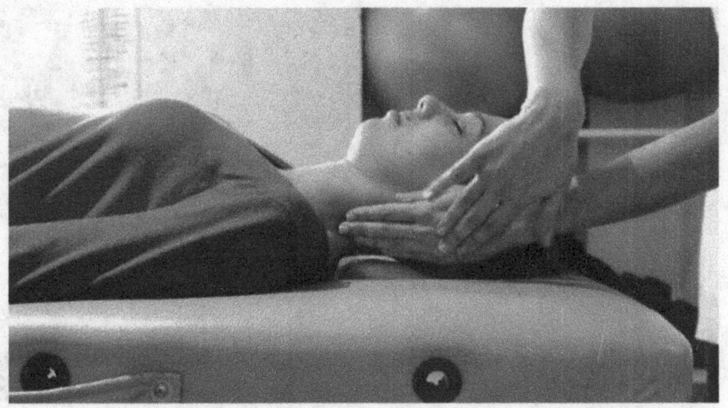

115. Cover the ear, and make a half-circle with your palm. Push your palm gently in order to create a "vacuum", and tap gently your hand with your fingers 2-3 times. Repeat at the other ear.

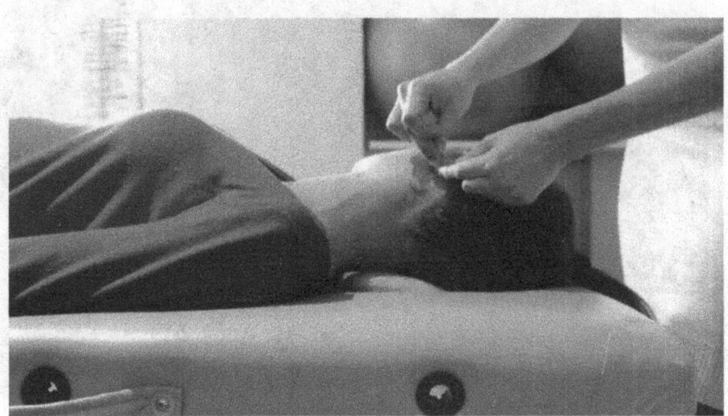

116. Rub and massage the earlobe. Repeat at the other ear.

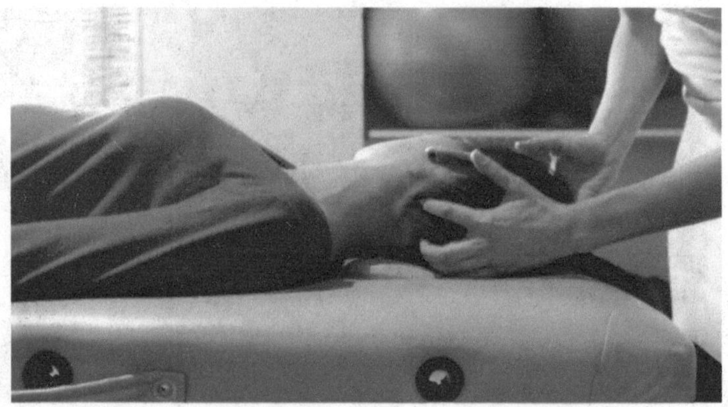

117. Shampoo the scalp – this is good for headaches. In order to do this properly, press your fingers firmly on the scalp, otherwise you will break the receiver's hair.

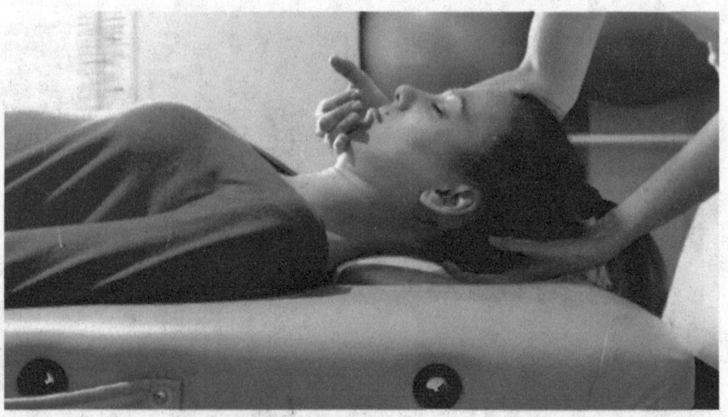

118. Grasp the atlanto-occipital joint, and with your other hand pull the head. Apply gentle pressure on the chin.

This concludes the face techniques.

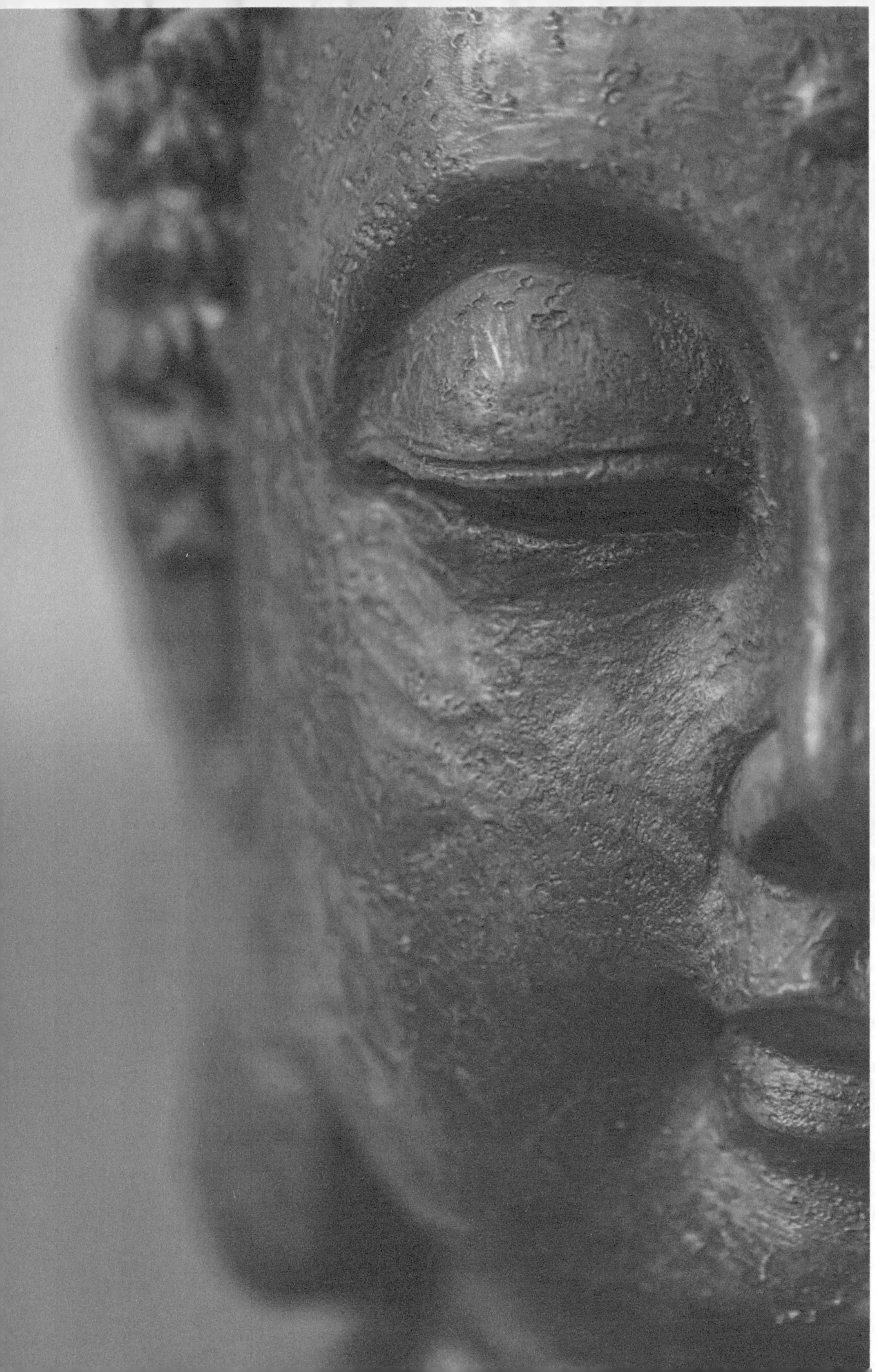

A few notes on the spine

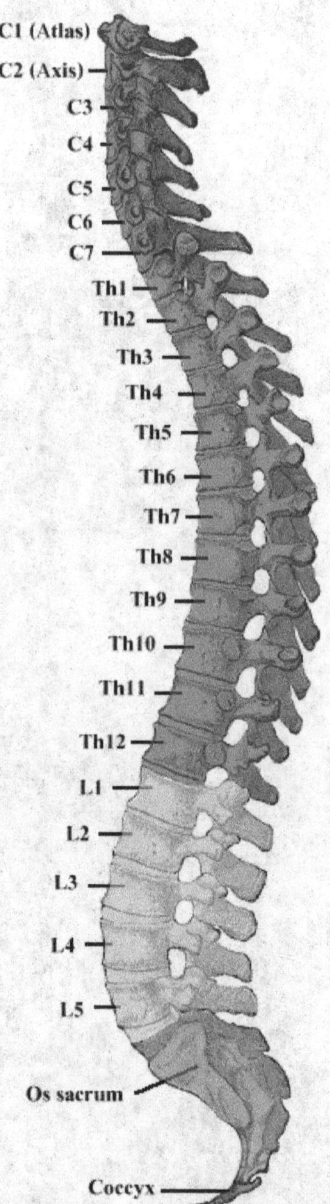

The spine, also known as vertebral column, is part of the axial skeleton.

Structure

In a human's vertebral column there are normally thirty-three vertebrae; the upper twenty-four are articulating and separated from each other by intervertebral discs, and the lower nine are fused in adults, five in the sacrum and four in the coccyx or tailbone. The articulating vertebrae are named according to their region of the spine. There are seven cervical vertebrae, twelve thoracic vertebrae and five lumbar vertebrae. The number of vertebrae in a region can vary but overall the number remains the same. The number of those in the cervical region however is only rarely changed.

There are ligaments extending the length of the column at the front and the back, and in between the vertebrae joining the spinous processes, the transverse processes and the vertebral laminae.

Vertebrae

The vertebrae in the human vertebral column are divided into different regions, which correspond to the curves of the spinal column. The articulating vertebrae are named according to their region of the spine. Vertebrae in these regions are essentially alike, with minor variation. These regions are called the cervical spine, thoracic spine, lumbar spine, sacrum and coccyx. There are seven cervical vertebrae, twelve thoracic vertebrae and five lumbar vertebrae. The number of vertebrae in a region can vary but overall the number remains the same. The number of those in the cervical region however is only rarely changed. The vertebrae of the cervical, thoracic and lumbar spines are independent bones, and generally quite similar. The vertebrae of the sacrum and coccyx are usually fused and unable to move independently. Two special vertebrae are the atlas and axis, on which the head rests.

Individual vertebrae are named according to their region and position. From top to bottom, the vertebrae are:

- Cervical spine: 7 vertebrae (C1–C7)
- Thoracic spine: 12 vertebrae (T1–T12)
- Lumbar spine: 5 vertebrae (L1–L5)
- Sacrum: 5 (fused) vertebrae (S1–S5)
- Coccyx: 4 (3–5) (fused) vertebrae (Tailbone)

Shape

The upper cervical spine has a curve, convex forward, that begins at the axis (second cervical vertebra) at the apex of the odontoid process or dens, and ends at the middle of the second thoracic vertebra; it is the least marked of all the curves. This inward curve is known as a lordotic curve.

The thoracic curve, concave forward, begins at the middle of the second and ends at the middle of the twelfth thoracic vertebra. Its most prominent point behind corresponds to the spinous process of the seventh thoracic vertebra. This curve is known as a kyphotic curve.

The lumbar curve is more marked in the female than in the male; it begins at the middle of the last thoracic vertebra, and ends at the sacrovertebral angle. It is convex anteriorly, the convexity of the lower three vertebrae being much greater than that of the upper two. This curve is described as a lordotic curve.

The sacral curve begins at the sacrovertebral articulation, and ends at the point of the coccyx; its concavity is directed downward and forward as a kyphotic curve.

The thoracic and sacral kyphotic curves are termed primary curves, because they are present in the fetus. The cervical and lumbar curves are compensatory or secondary, and are developed after birth. The cervical curve forms when the infant is able to hold up its head (at three or four months) and to sit upright (at nine months). The lumbar curve forms later from twelve to eighteen months, when the child begins to walk.

These curves increase the spine's resistance to vertical forces. In comparison to a hypothetical straight spine, this resistance is increased by ten times, thanks to these three main curves. Actually, the body's resistance is reinforced by the curves of the knees and the feet.

Curvature

Excessive or abnormal spinal curvature is classed as a spinal disease or dorsopathy and includes the following abnormal curvatures:

- Kyphosis is an exaggerated kyphotic (concave) curvature in the thoracic region, also called hyperkyphosis. This produces the so-called "humpback" or "dowager's hump", a condition commonly resulting from osteoporosis.
- Lordosis as an exaggerated lordotic (convex) curvature of the lumbar region, is known as lumbar hyperlordosis and also as "swayback". Temporary lordosis is common during pregnancy.
- Scoliosis, lateral curvature, is the most common abnormal curvature, occurring in 0.5% of the population. It is more common among females and may result from unequal growth of the two sides of one or more vertebrae, so that they do not fuse properly. It can also be caused by pulmonary atelectasis (partial or complete deflation of one or more lobes of the lungs) as observed in asthma or pneumothorax.
- Kyphoscoliosis, a combination of kyphosis and scoliosis.

Thai Table Massage and Pregnancy

Massage during pregnancy should be taught in a dedicated course. However, I will just mention a few guidelines for those of you who plan to attend a course, or have already attended one.

Contraindications

- It is better to avoid massage altogether during the first trimester. Although massage cannot affect a healthy pregnancy, it is always wise to avoid it in this phase for legality reasons.
- After the first trimester, the woman should be placed either in the side position, or in a semi-reclining position. Avoid the supine position, and of course the prone position.
- Herbal packs should not be used during pregnancy, as they are too hot.
- Avoid pressing (palm walking and thumb walking, etc.) the inner side of the legs, because during pregnancy there is a high tendency for the formation of blood clots there.
- During pregnancy, the hormone relaxin causes ligamentous laxity (in order to facilitate childbirth). Thus, it is inadvisable to apply dynamic stretches to a pregnant woman.
- Nausea can be triggered by strong smells even during the second trimester. The massage room should be well ventilated, and there should not be

any strong odors (like the ones from the Thai heat rubs).

Positioning

- Your massage table should be wide, if you plan to offer Thai Table to pregnant women.
- At the side position, place the thigh almost parallel to the table, using pillows, yoga bricks or special props. This ensures that the belly is not compressed. The arm should be also placed on props, so that the arm is parallel to the table. The woman's head should be properly supported with pillows.

Benefits

- Techniques that create space in the thoracic cage are usually beneficial, since many pregnant women suffer from dyspnea.
- Massage the shoulders and do light stretches, as most pregnant women suffer from upper back pain.
- As the center of gravity is transferred upwards, many pregnant women have lordosis and suffer from lower back pain. Be sure to create space at the lower back, and balance the area with correct mobilizations.
- Of course, you will not be able to massage the belly (even if you intended to, you just can't press it!). If the woman suffers from constipation, press the acupoint San Jiao 6 (it is located on the Itha and Pingkala arm branch).

With proper education, the techniques of Thai Table Massage can be very beneficial during pregnancy.

Intake form

The following questions can be used as an intake form.
Before offering any massage treatment, you should be
aware of the client's medical history. Keep this form, and be
sure to update it in case of any changes.
Feel free to copy and distribute this client intake form.

Name:
Phone:
Email:
Date of Birth:
Occupation:
Emergency Contact Phone:
Date of Initial Visit:

Please answer the questions to the best of your knowledge.

- Have you ever received Thai Massage, Thai Table
  Massage or manual therapy in the past? If yes, how
  many times?
- Do you have any difficulty lying on your front, back,
  or side?
- Do you remain in a seated position for long hours?
  If yes, where and how?
- Describe any repetitive movements you may be
  doing.
- Is there a particular area of the body where you are
  experiencing pain or discomfort?
- Do you have, to the best of your knowledge, spinal
  stenosis, or any degenerated discs? If yes, in which
  area of the spine?
- Do you have any allergies?

Please note any cardiovascular or respiratory conditions.

Are you taking any medication? If yes, please note it.

Do you have osteoporosis?

Are you pregnant? If yes, what is the estimated date of delivery?

Do you have any particular goals in mind for this massage session?

Is there anything else about your health history that you think your therapist should know?

The above information will allow us to offer you a safe treatment. Feel free to ask any questions about the information we request. All information will be kept confidential.

Therapist's name and signature

Client's name and signature

Crafting a Thai Table Massage session

I will give you some suggestions on how to craft a Thai Table Massage session. I use the word craft, because I consider it a kind of art.

In this book, I present a lot of mobilizations. Have in mind that if you apply all of them, or even many of them during a session, this will be tiring - and also unnecessary - for the receiver.

When you meet the client, you have to ask them some basic questions about their medical history (refer to the previous pages for an intake form). We are mainly concerned with issues on the musculoskeletal system, but we also need to know about any serious health problems. Be sure to ask the client about areas of discomfort, limited range of motion and also, about his or her expectations and goals from a Thai Table massage session.

I do not recommend "choreographies" and ready-made treatments. It is best to master many techniques for many problems, and apply them as needed. An experienced therapist will be able to compose a session in his mind in seconds, according to what he hears from the client.

I believe that a treatment should not last more than 60 minutes. You also have to decide the percentage of mobilizations. For example, I like to keep the percentage of strong mobilizations and passive stretching to 30% of the time of the session. The rest should be dedicated to kneading, work on the Sen lines and acupressure, and focused remedial techniques. Feel free to offer treatments that last 45 or even 30 minutes, if you think you can offer comfort to the client in this time.

Sometimes, a client may complain of neck pain, and state this as his main issue. However, the human body does not consist of isolated areas, and you will have to work on some seemingly remote areas, in order to balance a painful spot. For example, I always work on the diaphragm, because I believe that it is a critical spot for our emotional experiencing, for our breath, and also for the lymphatic drainage of the entire body. You may also have to work on the lower back, as tensions and imbalances in this area tend to affect the upper part of the back. You will have to explain to the client that you will not focus your work solely on the neck and shoulders, because you must balance the surrounding tissues as well. Before starting the session, give a very short description of the order of the techniques you plan to apply. If you fail to do this, the client may become nervous during the session, if e.g. he has asked you to work on his neck and you are doing techniques for the pelvis in the beginning of the session.

In any case, learn to listen to the tissues, and respect the limits they set. Observe the client's face for any facial expressions that show pain or discomfort, and ask for feedback in case you see something like that. On the other hand, keep verbal communication to a minimum, and allow the client to experience your work in silence, as much as possible.

Epilogue

I hope you liked this book. Please have in mind that it is a small budget production, and it was made mostly by one person – me!

The photos are actually screenshots from a video I created, which is released in Amazon as the DVD, Thai Table Massage. This video was shot in my massage school, Flow – Wellness & Training, in Athens, Greece. The model is a student who volunteered, in exchange for training.

May these techniques be useful for your practice. If you have not attended a course, I hope it will inspire you to learn some type of massage therapy and bodywork. This, I believe, is a sacred art, and it has a huge impact on one's character and life if practiced with sincerity and dedication.

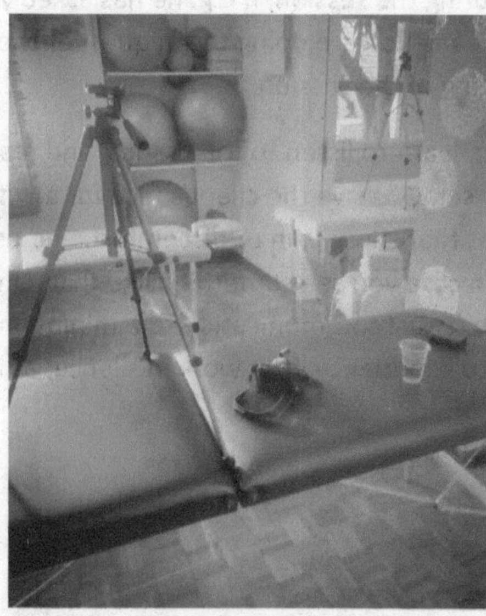

This is how we did it!

About the author

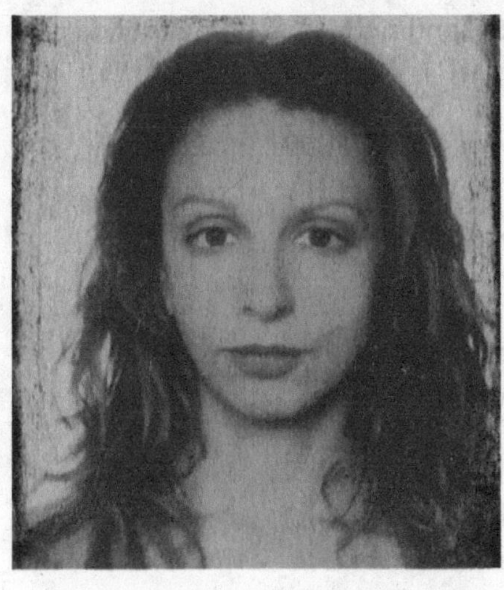

My name is Elefteria Mantzorou. I was born in Athens, Greece. From my childhood I felt attracted to herbal medicine and alternative treatments.

Disregarding any common sense, and following the flow of events without any conscious decisions, I found myself in Thailand many times. There, I studied Thai Massage, Thai Foot Massage & Thai Herbal Compress at the Old Medicine Hospital, and at the school of the unforgettable Mama Lek and her son Jack Chaiya. I also met personally Tai Chi instructor, Tew Bunnag.

For several years I lived as a backpacker. I went to many places in Europe and Asia, working as a volunteer, studying, staying in ashrams, or simply traveling. I worked as a volunteer in wildlife sanctuaries, and have treated countless wild animals. In these sanctuaries, I also worked as a surgeon's assistant.

Another experience that has remained indelible in my memory is my acquaintance with Masanobu Fukuoka and natural farming, as I had volunteered in one of his projects in Greece.

In between my trips, I studied alternative medicine (aromatherapy, herbal medicine, Swedish massage and anatomy, physiology and pathology) and was certified as a medical translator. I also attended courses on osteopathy. I started teaching in 2004, and since then I have trained hundreds of people.

In 2013 I opened my own school, FLOW, in a quiet neighborhood of Athens. Well, until I start travelling again, you might find me somewhere here:

FLOW - Wellness & Training
8, Milona str., 11363 Athens
Website: jointheflow.weebly.com

Facebook: Flow – Wellness and Training
Instagram: @FlowAthens
YouTube: Flow – Wellness and Training

Be always well!

Credits

All photos that demonstrate Thai Table Massage techniques, as well as the plates that depict Sen lines, constitute copyrighted property of Elefteria Mantzorou. Their non-authorized use will be persecuted.

The anatomy plates and descriptions are from Gray's Anatomy (taken from Wikipedia) and are in the public domain.

The traditional Thai meridian illustrations are reproduced with the kind permission of the British Library.

Design, text and artwork by Elefteria Mantzorou.